Praise for Jorge Cruise and *The Belly Fat Cure*

*"Jorge Cruise gets it right by eliminating excessive sugar and processed carbohydrates.
His recipes make eating smart easy. I recommend them highly."*

— **Andrew Weil, M.D.,**
Director of the Arizona Center for Integrative Medicine,
University of Arizona, and author of *Why Our Health Matters*

*"**The Belly Fat Cure** makes a solid case for healthful eating based on sound science. This way of
eating will increase your energy, help you slow the aging process, and reduce your risk for major
killers like heart disease and cancer. I strongly advise you to listen to Jorge's recommendations."*

— **Terry Grossman, M.D.,**
co-author of *Transcend: Nine Steps to Living Well Forever*

*"When it comes to your health, forward thinking will allow you to avoid obesity and disease and
achieve longevity. Jorge's program springs from progressive science that can truly change your
body—and it all starts with controlling your consumption of sugar and processed carbs."*

— **Ray Kurzweil,**
world-renowned scientist and author of *The Singularity Is Near,
When Humans Transcend Biology,* and *Fantastic Voyage: Live Long Enough to Live Forever*

*"Jorge, again, is on to something; belly fat is surely an indicator of poor health.
This book will turn your life around."*

— **Suzanne Somers,**
actress and best-selling author of *Breakthrough: Eight Steps to Wellness*

*"I put the Belly Fat Cure into practice and took 15 pounds off around my middle.
I obviously endorse this book!"*

— **Dr. Wayne W. Dyer,**
the #1 *New York Times* best-selling author of *Excuses Begone!*

"Like me, Jorge Cruise practices what he preaches."

— **Jack LaLanne,**
godfather of fitness and co-author of *Fiscal Fitness*

*"In this revelatory yet practical book, Jorge raises our awareness of innocent-seeming foods
that trigger insulin responses which keep us unwell and thick around the middle.
He then guides us to choose readily available and easily prepared substitutions, ensuring
that the solution to our hidden dependence on sweets will be as easy and delicious as it is healthy."*

— **Carol Brooks,**
Editor-in-Chief, *First for Women*

The

BELLY FAT
CURE™

The

BELLY FAT
CURE™

Discover the new **CARB SWAP SYSTEM**™
and lose 4 to 9 lbs. every week

JORGE CRUISE

HAY HOUSE, INC.
Carlsbad, California • New York City
London • Sydney • Johannesburg
Vancouver • Hong Kong • New Delhi

Published and distributed in the United States by: Hay House, Inc.: www.hayhouse.com • **Published and distributed in Australia by:** Hay House Australia Pty. Ltd.: www.hayhouse.com.au • **Published and distributed in the United Kingdom by:** Hay House UK, Ltd.: www.hayhouse.co.uk • **Published and distributed in the Republic of South Africa by:** Hay House SA (Pty), Ltd.: www.hayhouse.co.za • **Distributed in Canada by:** Raincoast: www.raincoast.com • **Published in India by:** Hay House Publishers India: www.hayhouse.co.in

Design: Charles McStravick
Cover and back cover photos: Jared Davis/JorgeCruise.com, Inc.

Notice: The information given here is designed to help you make informed decisions about your body and health. The suggestions for specific foods, nutritional supplements, and exercises in this program are not intended to replace appropriate or necessary medical care. Before starting any exercise program, always see your physician. If you have specific medical symptoms, consult your physician immediately. If any recommendations given in this program contradict your physician's advice, be sure to consult him or her before proceeding. Mention of specific products, companies, organizations, or authorities in this book does not imply endorsement by the author or the publisher; nor does mention of specific companies, organizations, or authorities imply that they endorse this book. The author and the publisher disclaim any liability or loss, personal or otherwise, resulting from the procedures in this program. Internet addresses and telephone numbers given in this book were accurate at the time it went to press.

Product pictures, trademarks, and trademark names are used throughout this book to describe and inform the reader about various proprietary products that are owned by others. The presentation of such pictures and information is intended to benefit the owner of the products and trademarks and is not intended to infringe upon trademark, copyright, or other rights; nor to imply any claim to the mark other than that made by the owner. No endorsement of the information contained in this book has been given by the owners of such products and trademarks, and no such endorsement is implied by the inclusion of product pictures or trademarks in this book.

Nutrition information for all brand-name products mentioned in this book was provided by company Websites or official nutrition labels. IHOP does not offer complete nutrition information to the public; therefore, the estimates for their meals were created from The Daily Plate (**thedailyplate.com**), owned by Demand Media, Inc., and **CalorieKing.com**, a service owned by Family Health Publications.

TRADEMARKS

The Belly Fat Cure	12-Second Sequence	Controlled Tension
The BellyFatCure.com	12Second.com	Jorge Cruise
Carb Swap System	3-Hour Diet	JorgeCruise.com
S/C Value	3HourDiet.com	Time-Based Nutrition
Body at Home	8 Minutes in the Morning	Jorge's Packs
	Be in Control	

Library of Congress Control Number: 2009932289

ISBN: 978-1-4019-2718-9
Digital ISBN: 978-1-4019-2762-2

13 12 11 10   11 10 9 8
1st edition, December 2009
8th edition, August 2010

Printed in China

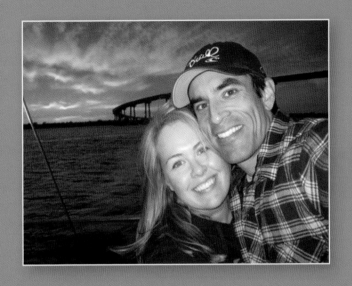

To Heather,
the woman who makes me
feel lucky every day.

Love,
Jorge

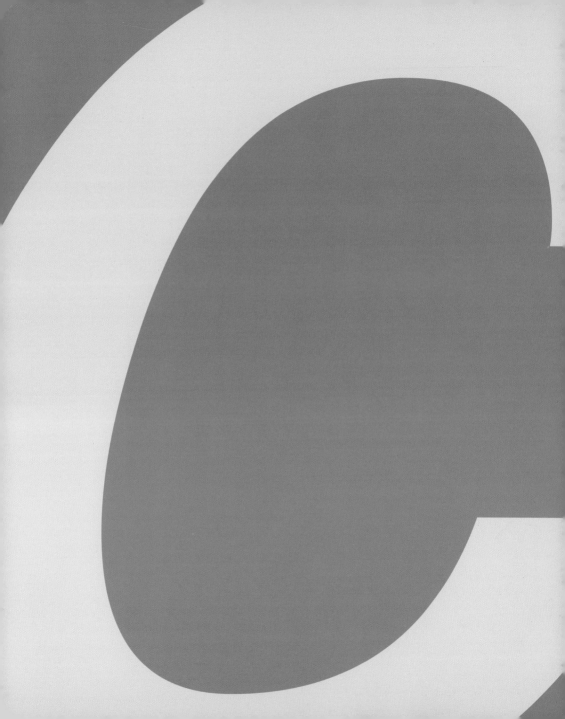

Contents

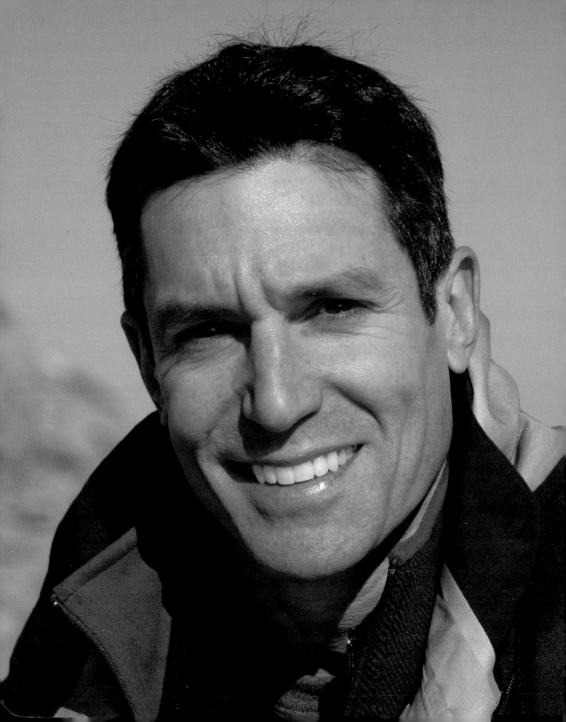

Dear Reader,

The ultimate solution to the threat of obesity is to "re-engineer" the modern environment so that eating well and being active each day are the societal norm, and the path of least resistance for us all. While many of us are working on that goal, I wouldn't recommend holding your breath!

What I *would* recommend instead is just what you are doing: reading this book. Because rather than waiting on the world to change, you can take matters into your own hands and change your lifestyle to control your weight and protect your health. And in that effort, you would be hard-pressed to find a more passionate, and compassionate guide, than my friend Jorge Cruise.

Jorge knows, as I do, that excess sugar in our diets is among the most important factors conspiring against our waistlines and our health. Too much sugar means increased risk of weight gain, obesity, hormonal imbalance, diabetes, heart disease, and even cancer. In *The Belly Fat Cure,* Jorge puts this threat in his crosshairs to help defend you from it.

Jorge knows about the challenge of weight loss and control, because he has confronted and overcome that challenge himself. And he knows that for guidance to be of any real use to you, you have to be able to follow it. In *The Belly Fat Cure,* Jorge offers his trademark variety of clear, kind, simple, supportive, real-world coaching. You can do this!

I commend you for being proactive in the defense of your health; it won't just take care of itself. For you to take care of it, a wise, kind, savvy, dedicated health coach would sure be helpful! That's just what you've found in Jorge Cruise.

With all best wishes,
David Katz, M.D., MPH, FACPM, FACP

Director and Co-Founder, Yale University Prevention Research Center;
Associate Professor, adjunct, of Public Health, Yale University School of Medicine;
Director & Founder, Integrative Medicine Center at Griffin Hospital;
Nutrition Columnist, *O, The Oprah Magazine*

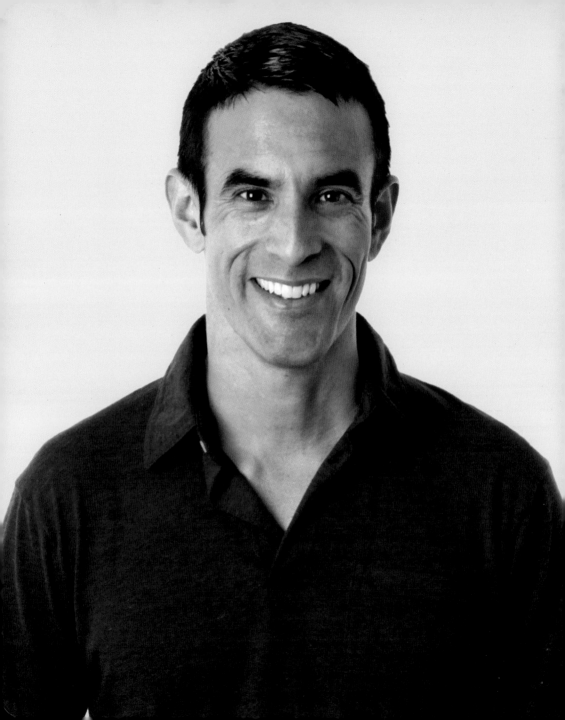

Dear Friend,

What if everything we've been told by conventional medical experts for more than 60 years was wrong? What if the truth on how to lose weight—especially from the waistline—has nothing to do with eating less or exercising more? This book is the culmination of a decade I spent answering these questions.

Not only is obesity taking over our world, in which 68 percent of us are overweight and sick, but this epidemic is bankrupting our economy with insane health-care costs numbering in the billions. Perhaps what's even more important is that being overweight also robs us of something even more essential if we want to live a truly extraordinary life: *confidence.* I know this because for most of my life I had belly fat, and every day I felt disempowered. The good news is that the science is clear—the smaller our waistlines, the more attractive we look and feel . . . and this directly enhances our confidence.

Imagine this: no dieting or exercising to lose weight. (Don't get me wrong—I love exercise, but I do it now only to build strength and endurance, not to lose weight.) With the Carb Swap System™, you'll discover the one simple key that never overstimulates production of insulin, the hormone that science proves pushes fat into fat cells. *Bottom line: you can't get fat if you keep your insulin under control.* This guidebook will actually steer you away from foods full of hidden sweeteners that deliver a belly-fattening sugar/carb value. So get ready to dig in and lose four to nine pounds a week.

Be well,

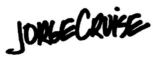

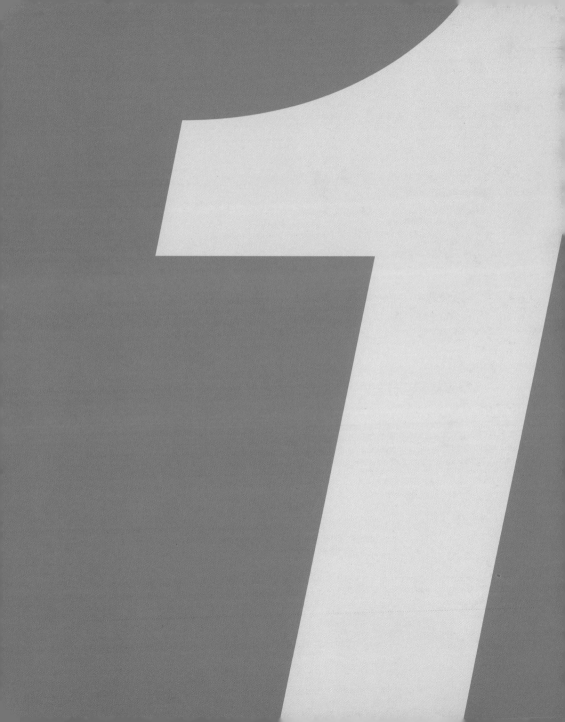

Lose Your Belly in
One Week!

"On the Belly Fat Cure", I lost an amazing 13 pounds in seven days and started feeling better about myself almost instantly. I have so much more energy and am motivated to go out and see my friends and be an active person. I wasn't even trying that hard and I lost that much weight—I'm amazed."

— **KAREN DIEGA SUTTON, lost 16 pounds**

What is the most important thing you can do to feel more empowered instantly? Lose belly fat. Nothing is as essential in changing how attractive you look. *Nothing.* **Study after study has confirmed that the less belly fat you have, the more attractive you will look.** There really is nothing more critical when it comes to looking truly attractive and feeling confident. How is it possible that this one thing can be so impactful? It's in our genes. For more than 160,000 years, we needed a method to help us in mate selection—and it was belly fat that allowed us to make a swift and accurate judgment of whom we would be attracted to in the most basic sense—for reproduction. So a high waist circumference meant a lack of health. And we knew automatically not to be drawn to people who had it.

I learned about this when I first interviewed my good friend Dr. Mehmet Oz, director of the Cardiovascular Institute at Columbia University Medical Center in New York and host of *The Dr. Oz Show* for my *USA WEEKEND Magazine* video blog. I will always remember that day. He was traveling outside of New York City and was at the West Coast Sony Studio lot as a guest on the game show *Jeopardy!* He and his production team had graciously invited my crew and me to film an interview for my readers at the studio. It was right there that we discussed this truth (he also writes about it in *YOU: Being Beautiful*) about the undeniable significance of one's waist measurement. According to research done at the University of Texas, waist circumference is the "first filter" people use to gauge someone's attractiveness—and it isn't just a superficial judgment, but rather, a deeply ingrained evolutionary adaptation. Additional research that appeared in the journal *Evolution and Human Behavior* confirmed waist circumference as an accurate indicator of attractiveness.

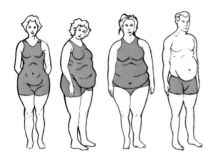

You see, in Paleolithic times, women needed to make sure a possible mate was healthy enough to have fertile sperm by having the right levels of testosterone (another visible indicator of enough testosterone was lean muscle development). What was the clearest sign of low testosterone? Belly fat. University studies done in Texas, Australia, and Sweden connected high levels of belly fat directly to low levels of available testosterone. Too much belly fat on a man converts testosterone to estrogen, which can lead to low sperm count and a lack of muscle. A woman's biological instincts would tell her that he wouldn't be a strong protector or provider, and most important, might not be a good reproductive partner.

The lead researcher from the University of Texas, Dr. Singh, explained it this way: "Waist-to-hip ratio [waist circumference], unlike stature, masculinity, and other signs of physical maturity, reliably signals present health status and future risk for various diseases and thus can be used as an indicator of mate quality." It was truly the fastest, most effective way to judge a mate's potential.

On the reverse side, if a male saw a protruding abdominal region on a woman, his instincts told him that she was either pregnant (off the market!) or could potentially have a hormonal imbalance, such as ovarian disease, which could cause infertility. Researchers at a prominent university in Spain and at the University of Wisconsin linked higher amounts of belly fat with polycystic ovarian disease and decreased fertility. Obviously, pregnancy or a perceived inability to get pregnant would make a man uninterested in a woman as a possible partner. Either way, a high waist circumference was a direct signal of a lack of health or availability.

So here's my first challenge to you: Stop feeling guilty about wanting to look good. It's hardwired in all of us. Most important, accept that being attractive on the outside means you are truly healthy on the inside.

Beauty Equals Health

With the Belly Fat Cure, the number one physical benefit you will experience almost immediately is increased energy. Belly fat has proven in studies to cause fatigue—a higher waist circumference can really zap your energy *and* your health. A research study done at Pennsylvania State University linked excess abdominal fat to increased levels of daytime sleepiness and overall fatigue. In another study, published in the *Journal of Clinical Sleep Medicine,* individuals with higher levels of belly fat were more likely to report feeling "exhausted" or "tired" than those with a healthy waist circumference. Belly fat is linked to causing sleep apnea, which severely disrupts sleep, leaving you constantly tired, and puts you at risk for other health problems and hormonal disturbances. This means that the moment you start losing abdominal fat with the Belly Fat Cure lifestyle, you will be on your way to renewed energy and vitality.

You will also begin to prevent free-radical damage, one of the main culprits in aging. Researchers at the Washington University School of Medicine in St. Louis confirmed that visceral belly fat (the kind that wraps around your internal organs, not the kind you can pinch) releases inflammatory molecules called interleukin-6; higher levels of these molecules are connected to increased levels of C-reactive protein, which in turn, is connected to chronic inflammation. Scientists in London substantiated this link by declaring visceral fat a "key promoter of . . . chronic inflammation." Even though inflammation starts out as our body's way to protect itself, when it becomes chronic, it causes cellular damage that ages our tissues and organs, and can eventually lead to arterial stiffness and heart disease. Beyond eliminating the damage that happens on the inside with the Belly Fat Cure, you will also slow down another outward sign of aging—wrinkles—something I know we'd all like to have fewer of!

On top of those benefits (not to mention the flatter stomach you'll see in one week), you will specifically lower your short-term *and* long-term risk for illness and disease. Perhaps most important of all, you will take a critical step toward preventing premature death. A groundbreaking research study published in November of 2008 in the *New England Journal of Medicine* revealed that losing belly fat was the most important determinant to a long life without disease. After tracking more than 350,000 Europeans for nine years, researchers determined that a high waist circumference doubled the risk of premature death.

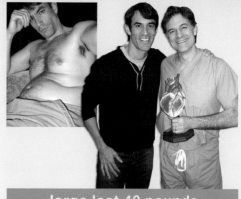

Jorge lost 40 pounds

Age: 38
Height: 6'1"
Pounds Lost: 40
Belly Inches Lost: 5

"I grew up with belly fat, and by the time I was a teen, my appendix burst and I almost died. Not long after, my father was diagnosed with prostate cancer and my grandparents passed away from heart disease. These experiences really defined my first health awakening—they're what got me on my path to health. Then a few years ago, I met Dr. Mehmet Oz (pictured with me above), who helped me understand how too much sugar was at the heart of the problem and a significant contributor to belly fat. This second awakening about sugar allowed me to make the connection to all of the health problems and disease in my family. At the time, we didn't know it was sugar, even though we were gorging on cakes and pies and giant bowls of Cap'n Crunch. Since then, I have never looked at sugar and belly fat the same—it has become my passion to educate other people about this dangerous connection."

BEST TIP FOR SUCCESS:

"Never miss breakfast; it's the most important meal of the day. My favorite meal for the morning is the Savory Breakfast Sandwich (sée recipe on page 65)."

In another study, researchers from Harvard Medical School determined that a higher waist circumference was linked to premature death in nearly 50,000 women.

Why is belly fat so dangerous to your health? It's directly connected to three of the biggest killers: heart disease, type 2 diabetes, and certain types of cancer (this is covered in greater detail in Chapter 2). This scary link is supported by medical experts from the Mayo Clinic and Harvard University. Belly fat has also been linked to additional health conditions such as chronic fatigue, sexual dysfunction, adrenal burnout, sleep apnea, premature aging, and immune disorders. Imagine erasing your concerns and fears of developing heart disease, type 2 diabetes, or cancer by simply losing belly fat. Your life will absolutely be renewed.

How It Works

When you lose 4 to 9 pounds from your waist a week on the Belly Fat Cure, not all of it will be from fat—only about 2 to 3 pounds will be from true belly fat. Where will the rest of the weight come from? The rest will be from what I call "false belly fat," which is simply trapped waste matter. As unpleasant as this may be to imagine, a lot of what may be giving you a high waist circumference is built-up waste in your intestines, the result of a lack of good carbohydrates in your daily diet. The fiber in good carbs is critical for removing this kind of waste from your body; the common diet of highly refined and processed carbs fails to "sweep" your intestines clean. You will experience the weight loss that's right for you (see the chart below). Your results will be dramatic, and you will look and feel revitalized!

Your Goal Total	Each Week
Lose 30 to 60+ lbs.	10 to 13 lbs.
Lose 10 to 29 lbs.	4 to 9 lbs.
Lose 3 to 9 lbs.	1 to 3 lbs.

Set Your Goals

Up until now, I have only talked about the weight you will lose when you follow the Belly Fat Cure, but most of the research I've mentioned confirms the importance of a different measure: your waist circumference. While stepping on the scale and confirming your weight loss is important (and the traditional way of "seeing" results), I also want you to measure your waist. In the past, medical professionals have measured health by looking at things such as: blood pressure, cholesterol levels, body mass index (BMI), and overall weight. Research has confirmed that, because how much abdominal fat you have is a key predictor of so many dangerous health conditions, it is an ideal way to measure your health. A study published by researchers at Harvard University revealed that even normal-weight individuals who still had belly fat were linked to increased health risks—making the waist measurement an equal or even better indicator of health than weight. Researchers in Canada said that a quick check of your waist circumference is "ideal as an inexpensive means" for predicting something as serious as heart disease—and all you have to do is wrap a measuring tape around your waist. **This is why my number one long-term goal for you is to ensure that you achieve and maintain a healthy waist circumference.**

Getting to that healthy measurement will also ensure that you remain attractive. According to the American Heart Association and the National Institutes of Health, if you're a woman, the goal should be 35 inches or less; if you're a man, the goal should be 40 inches or less. If you want to get more specific based on your height, take your height in inches and divide it by two—this will be your ideal waist circumference. For example, I am 6'1", which is 73 inches. If you divide that by two, you get 36.5 inches—this is my maximum ideal waist circumference.

How do you measure your waist? Grab a tape measure (you can pick one up at any drugstore) and suck in your belly as tight as you can—make sure to really suck it in. Measure your waist around your belly button, not too high or low. Visit **TheBellyFatCure .com** and join my free VIP e-mail club to get access to a video demonstration with Dr. Oz and me. This was one of the first videos I ever filmed with him, and it has become one of my most-watched videos on YouTube. Use the simple chart on the next page to enter your current measurements and your goal.

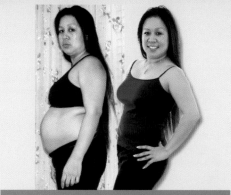

Karen lost 16 pounds

Age: 38
Height: 5'0"
Pounds Lost: 16
Belly Inches Lost: 4

"Before the Belly Fat Cure, my self-esteem had dropped so low that I stayed in most nights eating instead of going out. I was up to my pregnancy weight—without being pregnant—and I couldn't think of anything positive about myself. Then in just seven days, my whole life changed: I lost 13 pounds and started feeling better about myself almost instantly. I have much more energy and am motivated to go out and be an active person. I wasn't even trying that hard and I lost that much weight. My boyfriend and friends can't believe the difference they see in me!"

BEST TIP FOR SUCCESS:

"Stop thinking that you're never going to change—use the S/C Value and you'll be amazed by the improvements in your life!"

5

My current weight: _____

My current waist: _____

My goal weight: _____

My goal waist: _____

Guarantee Your Success

What is a simple thing you can do right now to ensure your success on the plan before you start? Establish a support network of people to help you on your health journey. I call this network of people your inner support team. This team can include family members, co-workers, and good friends— anyone whom you feel comfortable communicating with openly and honestly. People in your inner support team must be caring and nonjudgmental; they must be willing to listen to you and support you. Start by thinking of three people you'd like to invite into your inner support team. Below, list their names (just their names for now) in the blanks on the left:

Name & Contact Info: _____   Buddy Type: _____

Name & Contact Info: _____   Buddy Type: _____

Name & Contact Info: _____   Buddy Type: _____

Now I want you to "assign" each person a buddy type and write in that designation, along with his or her contact information, in the blanks on the right. Here are the types:

E-mail buddy. Designate one of the three people you listed as an e-mail buddy, and fill in his e-mail address in the contact-information area. Anytime you feel that you need to reach out for encouragement, send an e-mail to your buddy and tell him how you're feeling.

Phone buddy. Designate another of the three people as a phone buddy and fill in her home, work, and cell-phone numbers. This buddy will help you when you need immediate support.

Accountability buddy. The last buddy on your inner support team is your accountability buddy. This person will help you stay accountable for your weight-loss goal by talking to you for up to 15 minutes every night during your first week, preferably at the end of each day. Your accountability buddy should be someone whose lifestyle you admire— someone who is healthy and fit and can serve as a role model. Write your accountability buddy's contact information in the appropriate space.

If you need to find more buddies, visit **TheBellyFatCure.com** and join my online video coaching club. It's an easy way to get more support and meet people from all over who are following the plan. You can catch up with me there, too—I'm often leading live online meetings.

Start Today

Follow any of my five one-week plans in Chapter 3 and you will lose up to 13 pounds from your waist, have more energy than you've had in a long time, and look attractive in your clothes again. Continue living the Belly Fat Cure lifestyle, and you'll experience these benefits; plus, you'll give yourself the gift of long-lasting health. All of these benefits will allow you to feel self-confident and empowered.

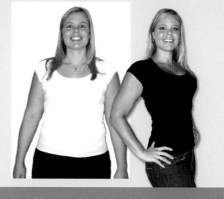

Dawn lost 20 pounds

Age: 37
Height: 5'7"
Pounds Lost: 20
Belly Inches Lost: 6

"I've tried everything (Atkins, The Zone, LA Weight Loss), only to gain the weight back, plus more! I have suffered from knee and back pain for years, probably due to being overweight. My weight had gotten to the point where it was hampering my social life. Jorge's program has been the easiest eating plan that I've ever tried! I have so much more energy, and I'm steadily losing weight. It's so easy, and I feel healthy and alive. I love this plan and have recommended it to many people I know. Thank you, Jorge! You have been my 'Aha!' moment."

BEST TIP FOR SUCCESS:

"Do not deprive yourself if you're hungry—grab a handful of nuts. They're filling and easy to haul around with you."

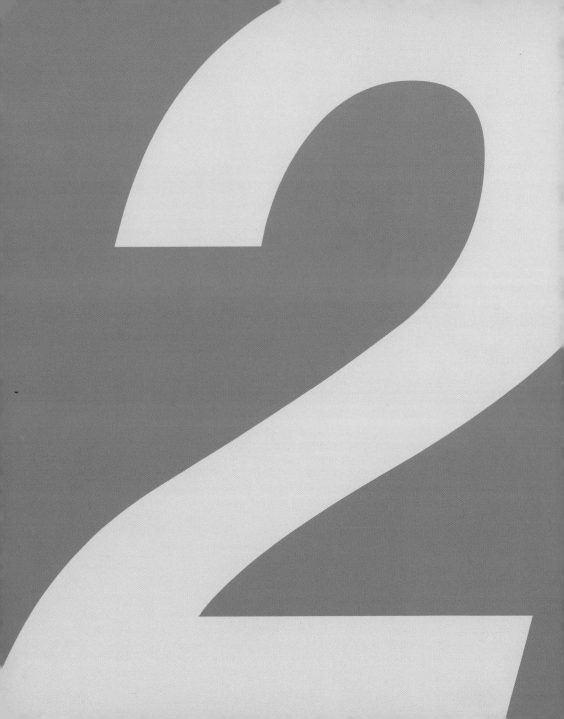

2 The One Critical Key

"The best part of the Belly Fat Cure lifestyle
for me is something much greater than just weight loss: the discovery
that excess sugar is dangerous to the immune system. I thought I was
eating healthfully and had no idea how much sugar was hidden in my
low-fat foods—I was eating upwards of 200 grams per day!"

— Michelle McGowen, lost 20 pounds

Now that you know what belly fat does to your body, you're probably ready to discover how to get rid of it. What I'm about to share with you
took me more than ten years to uncover. There is only one critical key to
getting rid of belly fat forever, and that is to lower insulin, the scientifically
proven hormone that pushes fat into fat cells. You see, you can't get fat or
stay overweight without insulin. This is a biological fact that was proven in
multiple research studies over the last 60 years that have appeared in such
respected publications as *The British Journal of Nutrition* and *The Journal
of the American Medical Association.* Unfortunately, this critical idea that
insulin is essential for storing fat—and lowering your insulin is essential for
releasing that fat—has been buried under the conventional medical com-
munity's message that it's all about calories in, calories out; that all you
have to do is exercise more and eat less to lose weight. It's a broken the-
ory; it's time for you to get ready for a new, intelligent, and effortless way
of eating.

The Carb Swap System™

The Carb Swap System is my trademarked eating method that guarantees that
you will automatically steer clear of foods full of the sweeteners and processed carbohydrates that chronically keep insulin levels high and belly fat present. The secret

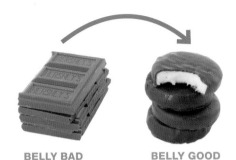

BELLY BAD **BELLY GOOD**

to the Carb Swap System is that it will ensure that you always hit what I have determined to be the magical sugar and carb values, or S/C Value™, each day. Write these two numbers down, since they're what all my work has revealed, and they will transform your body forever: 15/6. **This means that each day your total eating goal needs to be 15 grams of sugar and 6 servings of carbohydrates.** This combination is called your daily S/C Value.

How did I come up with 15 and 6? Well, the 15 grams of sugar a day was based on two things: First, in my research on the evolution of nutrition, it was evident that early humans didn't consume any sugar because it didn't exist (with the exception of honey and fruit), and it certainly didn't exist in the refined form it does today. Men and women dating back 40,000 years ago—we'll call them Stone Agers—ate only the foods that allowed their bodies to function at their best. During this time, almost everyone had an ideal body mass and didn't have diabetes, high blood pressure, or heart disease (of course, these Stone Agers had other scary things to worry about, like saber-toothed tigers). Researchers at Colorado State University confirmed that these early humans were "largely free" of diseases associated with modern societies.

Regardless of how drastic the changes have been to our diet since that time, our bodies aren't different . . . except for the fact that we cover them in clothes. According to research published in *The Journal of Nutrition,* genetically we haven't had time to adapt to a diet of highly processed, sugar-filled foods, which is why obesity and disease levels have reached an all-time high. This means that the absolute ideal would be to get back to a diet similar to the Stone Agers, but based on the reality of the foods available today, eating a no-sugar or no-processed-carb diet is virtually impossible. Instead, we should return to what researchers from the University of Toronto say was consumed for "thousands of years"—about 15 grams of sugar per day. Not only is 15 grams a day possible, it's enjoyable. How do I know this? Because my second reason for coming up with this amount is based on real tests with everyday people just like you. Fifteen grams has been client-tested and enthusiastically approved. My clients have found that this amount allows them to enjoy eating while eliminating belly fat fast. Remember, this is a lifestyle that will work for your busy, modern life. That's why I recommend about 5 grams of sugar per meal, for a total of 15 grams per day.

Why did I select six servings of carbs (about 120 grams) for you each day? Because it allows you to eat the carbs you love, but still keeps insulin levels low enough to lose your belly fat. A research study published in the *American Journal of Clinical Nutrition* revealed that participants who ate between four and seven servings a day of whole-grain, complex carbs lost significantly more weight from their abdominal region than those who got their carbs from refined sources. Aim for six servings and you will quickly start to shed your false belly fat.

With more than 100 easy, at-home Carb Swap meals in Chapter 4, there's no thinking involved—you just enjoy these meals for breakfast, lunch, and dinner and you'll never go over 15/6. Plus, you'll find more than 600 Carb Swap grocery products in Chapter 5 and more than 800 everyday food items in Chapter 6. Many of the items have pictures to make it even easier for you to know what to eat to lose belly fat.

I suggest that you learn how to apply the S/C Value to all of the foods you want to eat. This will allow you to calculate the S/C Value for any food you love and know if it's what I call a "Belly Good" or a "Belly Bad" item. You can skip this part if you want, but I strongly believe that having this understanding will help you make this plan a lifestyle. Here's how the S/C Value works; it's as simple as A, B, C:

A. Know your sugar. The first number (the "S") is the amount of sugar in any food represented in grams. Anything under .5 grams is not counted.

B. Know your carbs. The second number (the "C") is the amount of carbohydrates in any food represented in servings: 5 to 20 grams is 1 serving; 21 to 40 grams is 2 servings; 41 to 60 grams is 3 servings. Anything under 5 grams is not counted. **It's very important to be exact. For example, if you eat something that has 21 carbohydrate grams, you can't count it as "1" carb serving—it's "2" carb servings.**

C. Track it. Using the planner (see page 36), cross off one sugar box per gram consumed and one carbohydrate box per serving consumed. Once you've checked off all of your boxes, you've reached your daily limit.

On page 12 is an example using chips. The "S" arrow points to the sugar content, which is a 0. The "C" arrow points to the carbohydrate content, which at 17, is a 1 using the S/C Value. This means that a serving of Mission Tortilla Triangles has an S/C Value of 0/1.

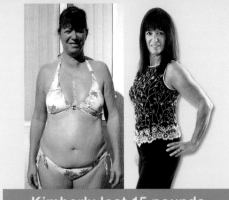

Kimberly lost 15 pounds

Age: 52
Height: 5'7"
Pounds Lost: 15
Belly Inches Lost: 6

"I was sick of having a fat belly, not looking nice in clothes, and constantly feeling tired. I always said that I'd never be overweight because of my mother, who spent the last five years of her life in bed with pain in her knees—they were unable to hold her weight. I have four kids, and I want to be around for a long time for them and my grandkids! I love this plan because it's easy to do, and I have more energy and am able to exercise with no problems. This program is so easy; it's the way I will eat for the rest of my life."

BEST TIP FOR SUCCESS:

"I take stevia or xylitol with me in my purse wherever I go."

Nutrition Facts

Serving Size 1oz (28g/about 10 chips)
Servings Per Package 14

Amount Per Serving

Calories 160   Calories from Fat 80

	% Daily Value*
Total Fat 9g	**14%**
Saturated Fat 4g	**20%**
Trans Fat 0g	
Cholesterol 0mg	**0%**
Sodium 150mg	**6%**
Total Carbohydrate 17g	**6%**
Dietary Fiber 1g	**4%**
Sugars 0g	
Protein 2g	

Vitamin A	0% • Vitamin C	0%
Calcium	2% • Iron	2%

*Percent Daily Values are based on a 2,000 calorie diet. Your daily values may be higher or lower depending on your calorie needs:

	Calories:	2,000	2,500
Total Fat	Less Than	65g	80g
Saturated Fat	Less Than	20g	25g
Cholesterol	Less Than	300mg	300mg
Sodium	Less Than	2,400mg	2,400mg
Total Carbohydrate		300g	375g
Dietary Fiber		25g	30g

Calories per gram:
Fat 9   •   Carbohydrate 4   •   Protein 4

Mission Tortilla Triangles
(10 chips)
S/C value ⓪/① 1

The rest of this chapter will focus on the science behind the Belly Fat Cure. You don't need a complete understanding of the facts to be successful, but any time I've shared the following information with my clients, they've experienced a profound "Aha!" moment. I want you to have this opportunity, too. What follows in two parts is the science of the Belly Fat Cure. Part I is about how too much sugar leads to belly fat. Part II is about how too few carbs leads to *false* belly fat.

PART I: How Too Much Sugar Leads to Belly Fat

Here's a fact: the average American consumes more than 47 teaspoons of sugar each day (this shocking number was revealed by researchers at Colorado State University); that's about 189 grams a day. About 200 years ago, daily consumption of sugar was under 15 grams—research has shown that before the Industrial Revolution, that's about how much the average person ate. Guess what you didn't see much of then? Belly fat. You also didn't see a population severely overwhelmed by obesity; compare that to now, where two-thirds of our population is overweight and sick and facing crippling medical bills due to the consequences of poor health habits. Don't get me wrong, I love sweets; but when you eat too much sugar, or what are technically called "caloric sweeteners" (sugar from cane or beet, corn syrup, fruit juice, or even milk), you develop belly fat in one primary way. Here's more on how it happens.

Increased Insulin

As I mentioned before, consuming sugar and refined carbs affects one of the most critical hormones in your body: insulin. Insulin is produced by your pancreas to manage your blood sugar and control the accumulation of fat—especially around your waistline. According to Nobel prize–winning physicist Rosalyn Yalow, co-inventor of the first accurate test used to measure insulin in the bloodstream, insulin is the "the primary regulator of fat tissue." Increased levels of insulin will make you fat and make sure you *stay* fat.

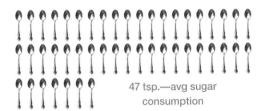

47 tsp.—avg sugar consumption

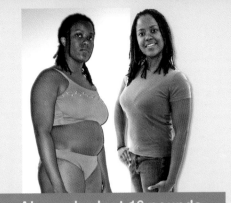

Alexandra lost 16 pounds

Age: 32
Height: 5'1"
Pounds Lost: 16
Belly Inches Lost: 6.5

Research published in *The European Molecular Biology Organization Journal* determined that insulin is probably the most important hormonal factor influencing the creation of fat, or what is scientifically called *lipogenesis.* In the book *Transcend,* my friends Ray Kurzweil and Dr. Terry Grossman used a scary visual to describe what happens to your blood when you consume too much sugar and it gets converted into fat—they suggested that your blood actually turns into a "pink cream." Imagine the most vital fluid in your body turning to a gooey glob that can barely get through your veins (yes, this can lead to problems other than belly fat—namely, high blood pressure and increased risk for heart disease and type 2 diabetes). If you're a healthy person, this fat in your blood may filter out in a few hours, but if you have diabetes or are prediabetic, it could linger in your blood even longer—or never go away. Even in healthy individuals, this fat still has to go somewhere, and it's most likely going to get deposited in abdominal fat cells. High levels of triglycerides have been connected to dangerous belly fat by researchers affiliated with the American Heart Association and the Mayo Clinic.

Once the fat in your blood (otherwise known as triglycerides) gets locked into your fat cells, they actually have to be broken down before they can move out and become usable energy. Insulin plays an important role here as well by preventing the triglycerides from breaking down—it wants to make sure that the fat stays put. And it does. Only when

"Before this plan, I had completely given up on myself. No amount of exercise or dieting gave me results. I was depressed; as well as suffering from acne, fatigue, and painful headaches. I was so ashamed of myself—I used to be an athlete, and I thought I knew a lot about nutrition. When I stumbled upon Jorge's program, I felt a little spark of hope—I'm amazed every day by how easy it is. I feel great, and I'm starting to look like my old self. I'm now motivated, I'm going out with friends again, and I have my smile back."

BEST TIP FOR SUCCESS:

"Plan ahead.
I make five sandwiches on Sunday
to get me through the week.
Sunday is also when I wash and
chop vegetables and defrost chicken
and fish for the week."

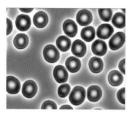

BEFORE SUGAR

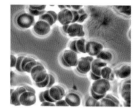

AFTER SUGAR

insulin disappears for a while can this fat escape from the cell to be used. **That's the primary way stored fat is released—your insulin levels absolutely have to be low.**

What's vitally important to understand is that not all foods trigger the same type of insulin response. Fats and proteins, for example, don't ever significantly drive up your insulin level (which, like I mentioned, is why we don't track them on this plan). Sugar and processed carbs, on the other hand, cause a rapid and dramatic increase in insulin levels, which directly causes your body to store fat. Sugar consumption can also lead to a condition known as "insulin resistance," which by itself drives up insulin levels and keeps them up. Various breakthrough studies done at Harvard University over the past decade have clearly shown that the main reason you have "belly fat" is that you've been eating too much sugar and processed carbohydrates, which keep your insulin levels chronically high—not because you've been eating too much fat or protein. It's that simple. To paraphrase George Cahill, a former professor of medicine at Harvard and an expert on insulin, "Carbohydrates [sugars] is driving insulin is driving fat." Does this mean you can eat a whole cow or ten sticks of butter because it won't trigger insulin production? No. You need to use common sense—but the good news is that proteins and fats satiate your hunger fast, so it's almost impossible to overeat them. As you'll see with all of my Carb Swap meals, my top pick for proteins are almost always lean meats. My top picks for fats are those that come from egg yolks, raw butter, extra-virgin olive oil, flax oil, or fish oil—and never dangerous hydrogenated oils.

I hope that by now you can see how important the hormone insulin is to regulating fat accumulation and to the Belly Fat Cure. When you eat using the Carb Swap System, you'll ensure that you keep your insulin response low. Plus, the great news is that once you begin to lose belly fat, you will actually improve your body's response to insulin and will have perfectly controlled fat regulation. Bottom line: to lose belly fat, you must keep your insulin levels low. Since sugar and carbs have the biggest impact on insulin, we only track sugar and carbs on the Belly Fat Cure—it's that simple, and it's the only way you'll lose weight. Like my mentor and good friend Gary Taubes, author of the groundbreaking *Good Calories, Bad Calories,* put it: "The only non-pharmaceutical remedy [to obesity] is to restrict or remove the cause—sugar and refined carbohydrates."

One Other Problem: Less Leptin

Another side effect of eating too much sugar is that you're programmed to overeat and gain belly fat. Why? While sugar drives up insulin production, it fails to trigger another hormone in your body that helps control appetite: leptin. Without enough leptin, your "signaling center" breaks down, and you quickly end up with a traffic jam of food in your body ready to get stored as fat. Where this fat gets

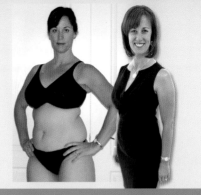

deposited depends on your genetics, but most of us start storing it in our midsection. Research published in the *American Journal of Clinical Nutrition* confirmed that foods sweetened with fructose, sucrose, glucose, and high-fructose corn syrup all have the same effect on leptin—they fail to produce it. Another study done at the University of California, Los Angeles (UCLA), discovered the same about lactose (milk sugar).

What happens when you don't have leptin? Research at the Albert Einstein College of Medicine in New York showed that when leptin was produced, it directly contributed to a decrease in abdominal fat. Without the right amounts of leptin, your body is programmed to store fat in your abdominal region. The most revealing studies were published in *The Journal of Clinical Endocrinology & Metabolism* and the *Annals of the New York Academy of Sciences,* which showed that the proper levels of leptin decreased abdominal fat by 32 percent and an extraordinary 62 percent, respectively. Making sure your diet contains foods that will regularly stimulate leptin production is essential to belly fat loss. These include proteins, fats, and complex carbs, which trigger leptin and make sure you're not set up to overeat.

Too Much Sugar Can Kill You, Too

Belly fat is what I would call the "physical marker" of eating too much sugar—it's the exterior consequence of a highly refined, processed diet filled with sweets, sodas, and nutrient-lacking foods. But sugar's damage goes beyond this and has been linked to three of the most deadly health conditions that may not have any exterior signs . . . until it's too late:

THE ONE CRITICAL KEY

Michelle lost 20 pounds

Age: 46
Height: 5'7"
Pounds Lost: 20
Belly Inches Lost: 7

"On this plan, I didn't think I'd lose much since I was able to still eat chocolate and ice cream, but after just *one* week, I was astounded by a seven-pound loss! Now I feel trim and have tons of energy. The best part for me, though, is something much greater: the discovery that excess sugar is dangerous to the immune system. After beating stage IIIB breast cancer, I thought I was eating healthfully. I had no idea how much sugar was hidden in my low-fat foods—I was eating upwards of 200 grams per day!"

BEST TIP FOR SUCCESS:

"Bake several chicken breasts at a time and keep them in the refrigerator. They can be sliced up and used in Caesar salads, nachos, or quesadillas."

1. Cardiovascular Disease: More Than 600,000 Annual Deaths

Sugar consumption has been linked to something called metabolic syndrome. This syndrome is a combination of a number of health conditions, including abdominal obesity, high cholesterol, high blood pressure, insulin resistance, and inflammation. Researchers at the University of Florida considered sugar to have a "major role" in igniting the health problems listed under the metabolic syndrome. One of the most dangerous aspects of the metabolic syndrome is inflammation, because this internal "swelling" is associated with arterial stiffness and heart disease. Inflammation causes your arteries to "swell in" and cause problems in circulation. To make matters worse, if you've been feeding your body a diet of sugar and refined carbs, those same arteries will begin to fill up with LDL, or "bad" cholesterol. To help attack the inflammation, your body responds by sending in white blood cells—but this attack actually releases toxic infection fighters that eventually land on your arteries, creating holes. These holes fill up with platelets and essentially scab over, adding even more and more buildup. The combination of these events leads to heart disease, which can result in a fatal heart attack.

One study, published in *Circulation,* the journal of the American Heart Association, confirmed that sugar intake is connected to increased triglyceride levels, a "known risk factor for coronary heart disease." Another research study conducted at the Harvard School of Public Health found that drinking two sodas a day (78 grams of sugar) increases your risk of heart disease by 35 percent. But there is a simple way to lower your risk (find out what soda I recommend on page 291—it has *zero* sugar).

2. Cancer: More Than 550,000 Annual Deaths

You probably know that when you have a weakened immune system, you're more susceptible to getting sick. But what you may not know is that this sort of shutting down of your defenses can lead to something much more serious than just a cold: cancer. Research done in Sweden linked excess sugar consumption to one of the most dangerous types of the disease, pancreatic cancer. They found that those individuals who consumed more sodas and foods with added sugars were more likely to get this tough-to-beat form of cancer. Another study published in the Journal of the National Cancer Institute revealed a link between colon cancer and sugar consumption. Research in Italy "found a direct association between breast cancer risk and consumption of sweet foods." Pretty scary. You see, sugar feeds cancer cells, helping them reproduce faster. Cancer cells love glucose, which is what your body breaks food down into so that it can be used as fuel. Even though all carbs convert to glucose, sugars and refined carbs provide the biggest rush of glucose into the blood, which cancer cells eagerly devour. When it comes to breast cancer, the increased risk is thought to also be related to the overproduction of insulin caused by sugar because insulin can stimulate the growth of cancerous cells in the breast.

3. Type 2 Diabetes: More Than 70,000 Annual Deaths

Speaking of the overproduction of insulin . . . you should know that this is one of the main factors that can lead to type 2 diabetes. When you eat foods loaded with sugar, your body produces extra insulin so that it can unlock cells and your body can use it for fuel. This is usually followed by a drop in blood sugar, which reignites the craving for more sugary foods. What's created is a vicious cycle that wears out your cells—so much so that they can eventually forget how to respond to insulin. This is what is known as insulin resistance, and once you have this, you're well on your way to type 2 diabetes. A Harvard study confirmed the link between consumption of sugars and increased risk of diabetes. Did I mention that excess sugar also leads to belly fat, which essentially ensures you're on the fast track to type 2 diabetes?

Research published in the journals of the American Heart Association and the American Diabetes Association described how visceral fat can begin to dump fatty acids and hormones directly into the liver, which causes it to produce too much glucose. Again, your body starts producing more insulin to try to manage the glucose. This cycle causes your body to become insulin resistant, which leads to type 2 diabetes. You see, even when your body's response to insulin is broken, your pancreas will continue to produce it to make sure that your body is getting fuel, and this simply wears your pancreas out. When your pancreas no longer produces enough insulin, or your cells fail to respond to insulin, you've reached the diabetic state. When you have diabetes, you're at risk for a long list of complications. According to the American Diabetes Association, you're susceptible to vision loss, kidney disease, circulation problems, skin problems, depression, nerve damage, gum disease, heart disease, and stroke. This means that although fewer people die from diabetes than the other two big killers, life expectancy *is* cut short in those with type 2 diabetes—by almost 15 years.

In addition, too much sugar can be responsible for premature aging and compromised immune health:

Aging. In Chapter 1, I briefly mentioned another nasty side effect of sugar (as if all of these terrible health risks and diseases aren't bad enough):

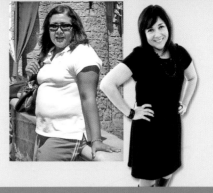

Marian lost 42 pounds

Age: 43
Height: 5'5"
Pounds Lost: 42
Belly Inches Lost: 6

"Doing the Belly Fat Cure was a life-changing experience and the best thing I've ever done regarding my health. I feel like Jorge gave me myself back. Today, I am 42 pounds lighter and have more energy. On top of that, my thyroid medicine has been decreased. Year after year, I've always been told that I have to take more medicine for my thyroid problem—now I'm taking less! I firmly believe that this is something my family and I could do for the rest of our lives. It's easy, and best of all, it works! Thanks, Jorge!"

BEST TIP FOR SUCCESS:

"Be creative with your meals
so you don't get bored.
Plus, enjoy treats—I ate blackberries
with whipped cream every day
on this plan."

wrinkles. I know that I said belly fat was really the main physical marker—and it's certainly the most dangerous one—but sugar won't stop there. Sugar in your bloodstream can also attach to the proteins there and create modified proteins called *advanced glycosylation end products,* or *AGEs* for short. Research published in *The Journal of Nutrition* recently confirmed the link between excess consumption of sugars and higher amounts of AGEs. The more AGEs you have, the faster actual aging processes occur in your body. These modified proteins can damage other proteins that perform important functions. Two of the most susceptible are collagen and elastin, which also happen to be essential to keeping your skin smooth and tight. Bottom line: your sugar consumption will begin to show itself in the very lines on your face. This is yet another reason to stick to no more than 15 grams of sugar a day.

Immune health. When you fill your body with sugar, you put your immune system in a weakened state. It actually impairs your immune system by not allowing your white blood cells to work properly. A study done by researchers at Loma Linda University in Southern California determined that "sugars impaired the neutrophils to engulf bacteria." Neutrophils are the main type of white blood cell you have in your body, and one of their main jobs is to gobble up bacteria and viruses that enter your body; sugar essentially wears them out so that they can't get that critical job done. If you ever feel like you're coming down with something, cut out sugar to help keep your defenses strong, get extra sleep, and take olive leaf complex. Olive leaf extract has one of the highest antioxidant values and helps support a healthy immune system.

Alternative Sweeteners: Not So Sweet

Now you may be thinking that the solution is to use alternative sweeteners, right? Nope. There are five sweeteners that I suggest you watch out for: **saccharin (pink packets), aspartame (blue packets), sucralose (yellow packets), high fructose corn syrup,** and **agave nectar.** The first three are known as excitotoxins, which contain neurotransmitters that "overexcite" neurons in the brain, causing degeneration and even death in these critically important nerve cells. I avoid these as much as possible and suggest you do the same. Here's more on these alternative sweeteners, along with two others I recommend you avoid:

Saccharin is the oldest sugar substitute around; you probably know it as Sweet'N Low. It was discovered by a chemist in 1879 and became a popular additive in the 20th century. As early as 1911, though, there was already an effort being made to ban it due to its potentially unhealthy effects. Controversy continued to follow saccharin, especially in the 1970s when research published in *Science* linked it to bladder cancer in animals. Again, there was an attempt to have it banned, but instead, products were required by law to post a label stating that saccharin caused cancer in laboratory animals (you probably remember seeing it on the side of popular sodas like Tab). Even though the ban has since been removed, scientists from institutions such as the University of Illinois and Boston University have requested that saccharin be labeled a carcinogen once again, stating that there is "ample evidence" to suggest it's cancer causing. I don't know about you, but if something has been proven to cause cancer in any living being, I don't want it in my body! It's not a risk I'm willing to take, which is why I avoid saccharin.

Aspartame was also discovered by a chemist; you probably know it as Equal and NutraSweet. It's found in thousands of food and drink products—namely, diet sodas. Studies have shown that it can cause imbalances in your brain; aggravate migraines; and affect your nervous system, your moods, and even your quality of sleep. A study published in *Environmental Health Perspectives* found a connection between aspartame consumption and seizures. Additionally, researchers from Washington University School of Medicine in St. Louis questioned the rise in malignant brain tumors during the years after aspartame was introduced.

Sucralose is found in more than 4,500 products on supermarket shelves, including Splenda. Also discovered by chemists, this sugar alternative is 600 times sweeter than sugar. Scientists at Duke University recently revealed that commonly consumed amounts of sucralose reduce the amount of "good" gut bacteria by 50 percent. Gut bacteria are essential for promoting a healthy digestive system and regular bowel movements, which help you get rid of false belly fat. Sucralose also produced significant weight gain in the study. Beyond this research, sucralose contains chlorine, which, as you know, is used to sanitize pools and is certainly not something you want to ingest. Manufactured chlorine compounds, like the ones used in Splenda, can cause damage to your organs and reproduction functions.

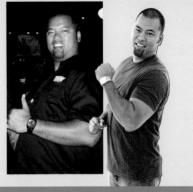

Ronald lost 20 pounds

Age: 40
Height: 5'11"
Pounds Lost: 20
Belly Inches Lost: 3

"I have a family history of high cholesterol, high blood pressure, and diabetes. In my late 30s, I went to a doctor's appointment and was told that I too had high blood pressure and high cholesterol and was on my way to getting diabetes. I was put on two medications and started working out, and slowly I did lose some weight. I could never get below 205 pounds, though, until I tried the Belly Fat Cure. The biggest change for me is learning about my sugar intake. Now I feel as healthy as ever, and my blood pressure and cholesterol are back to normal!"

BEST TIP FOR SUCCESS:

"Enjoy a hearty breakfast that gives you energy straight through the morning. Realize that every day is a chance to improve."

High-fructose corn syrup (HFCS) is something you've probably heard is bad for you, but you might be confused about *why* it's so bad. All simple sugars that enter the bloodstream can cause a rapid increase in blood sugar, but fructose has a specific effect on your body—and it's not a good one. Fructose has also been linked to leptin resistance, kidney stones, nonalcoholic fatty liver disease, diabetes, metabolic syndrome, and heart disease. When you consume fructose, it goes directly to your liver and gets processed into fatty deposits, which can lead to fatty liver disease—which is typically seen only in alcoholics. This fat also filters into your blood and fills your veins with fatty blood, otherwise known as high cholesterol. Since the introduction of HFCS into mainstream foods in the '70s, the American obesity epidemic has skyrocketed. If you track the rise in obesity and the rise in consumption of HFCS, you'll almost see a direct parallel. To make matters worse, high-fructose corn syrup has invaded nearly all types of food—you can find it in breads, sodas, juices, pastas, baking ingredients, cookies, ice cream, sauces, salad dressings, jellies . . . just about everything. According to the USDA, the availability of HFCS has increased 10,673 percent since 1970 (yes, you read that number right).

Agave nectar is a sweetener made from the agave plant, a common succulent found in Mexico. It's a bit like honey, but thinner. It's been labeled a healthy sweetener and said to be good for diabetics and "100 percent natural." But here's why it's landed on my list of wrong sugars: it is actually highly processed and has even more fructose in it than high-fructose corn syrup—agave nectar can be up to 90 percent fructose. According to Dr. Ingrid Kohlstadt, a fellow of the American College of Nutrition, "It's almost all fructose, highly processed sugar with great marketing." And Dr. Joseph Mercola, author of *Sweet Deception: Why Splenda®, NutraSweet®, and the FDA May Be Hazardous to Your Health,* says that "agave nectar is neither a natural food nor organic." Don't believe the hype and the labels that claim this to be a "healthy" alternative to sugar. It will actually trigger the same responses as white sugar and high-fructose corn syrup. I recommend avoiding it entirely—my personal doctor believes that it's worse than any other sweetener available!

Smart Sugar

So what can you eat that's sweet? The most critical thing you can do is to make sure you stick to 15 grams of sugar or less per day. If you make smarter choices about sweetness, you can still indulge your sweet tooth if you have one. (See page 267 for smart options.) My top recommendations for a healthy "real sweet" taste are stevia and xylitol. These are categorized as "nutritional supplements," and you can find them at all health-food stores or even online at **TheBellyFatCure.com**.

Stevia is an herb that originated in South America; it contains no calories, does not cause blood-sugar spikes, and can be used in baking. It's much sweeter than sugar, which means that you need only a little bit to get the right amount of sweetness. Recently, stevia was approved by the FDA for use in food and drink products, and it's the first herb-based sweetener to get that approval. Research published in the journal *Life Sciences* and in the *Journal of Human Ecology* revealed that stevia is effective in reducing blood pressure and hypertension. Turn to page 308 for more info on the types of stevia I recommend. My favorite soda, Zevia, uses Stevia (see page 291 for more information).

Sugar alcohols are considered nonnutritive sweeteners—this means that they add sweetness to foods and drinks without any nutrients and virtually no calories. Registered dietitians with the Yale-New Haven Hospital confirmed that sugar alcohols have fewer calories than sugar. They also revealed another benefit: these sweeteners don't cause cavities. Contrary to their name, sugar alcohols are neither a sugar nor an alcohol, but rather, a type of carbohydrate. The reason they have fewer calories is that they aren't completely absorbed by the body (most of consumed sugar alcohols will be excreted in urine). They also don't cause blood-sugar spikes like regular sugar does, which means they cause less disturbance to the endocrine system.

There are several types of sugar alcohols, but some of the most popular are xylitol, erythritol, and maltitol. On the Belly Fat Cure, we don't count any grams listed as "sugar alcohols" in the sugar category. However, they may be counted on a label under "total carbohydrates," which means that they'll be counted as carbs in the S/C Value (but you won't have to track these separately). Because sugar alcohols are incompletely absorbed, some can cause gas and bloating when eaten in excess; for this reason, you should avoid eating more than 100 grams in one day. Here's a little more about the sugar alcohols you're most likely to encounter:

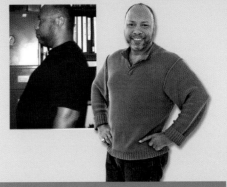

Duke lost 18 pounds

Age: 48
Height: 5'10"
Pounds Lost: 18
Belly Inches Lost: 10

"With the signs of aging and low self-esteem, I knew that it was time to get back into the gym. I started walking, yet I yo-yoed for several months. Then I tried my doctor's recommendation to reduce fats and calories; that didn't work either. Now everything is simple. This program has helped me shave almost $225 off of my monthly food bill as well. With the Belly Fat Cure, I haven't felt bloated, I feel lighter, my posture is better, and I sleep better, too. I know that my energy is up, along with my sex drive. Yes, that's right, sex drive! Thanks, Jorge."

BEST TIP FOR SUCCESS:

"Get your family and friends on your side. Let them know what you're doing. They will help you."

Xylitol is a sugar alcohol derived from the fiber of various fruits and vegetables. It was originally extracted from birch trees and was found in research done in Finland to help prevent the advancement of osteoporosis.

Maltitol has become very popular for use in baked goods, chocolates, and cookies. Having said that, some of my clients have discovered that too much maltitol can make them feel bloated. Although the reaction is harmless, you may want to adjust your intake of foods that contain maltitol based on your reaction to them.

Erythritol is one of the best sugar alcohols to look for. Research published in the *British Journal of Nutrition* revealed that it causes significantly less intestinal disturbances. In fact, the fermentation that can occur when other sugar alcohols are consumed in excess does not occur with erythritol—this just means it's less likely to cause gas.

PART II: How Too Few Carbs Leads to "False" Belly Fat

The second part of the belly fat problem is not eating enough of the right kind of carbohydrates, which are a key source of *fiber* that moves out hardened waste matter. Many carbohydrates have a more complicated "fibrous" structure, which makes them break down more slowly in your body, and chances are you aren't eating enough of them. Here's the bottom line: carbs are truly the only source of fiber. The right kind of carbs can eliminate any "false belly fat" that may come from built-up waste in your intestines and colon. Ideally, you should be having one to three healthy bowel movements a day. If you're eating enough fiber, you shouldn't have a problem with your body cleansing itself naturally. If you're not going to the bathroom enough, you might have one of those firm, hard bellies that sticks out. That's from built-up waste in your intestines. You've got to get rid of that false belly fat! By eating three Carb Swap meals each day, you'll be getting close to my ideal goal for you, which is 25 to 30 grams of fiber a day. I even have a Belly Fat Cure drink on page 101 that will give you 10 grams of fiber at one time to help you boost the flushing of false belly fat.

When you eat six servings of carbohydrates per day, you will ensure false belly fat loss. As I mentioned in the beginning of the chapter, research published in the *American Journal of Clinical Nutrition* revealed that participants who ate between four to seven servings a day of whole-grain complex carbs lost significantly more weight from their abdominal region than those who got their carbs from refined sources. Research giants Harvard University and the Mayo Clinic praise complex carbs for their belly-reducing benefits; they both suggest increasing complex-carbohydrate intake over refined or simple carbs specifically to reduce dangerous visceral fat. At the University of South Carolina, researchers established the same relationship between complex carbs and belly fat—they discovered that consuming foods with fiber was directly linked to losing belly fat. This means that you should aim to get most of your six carb servings a day from complex carbohydrates. This will help you get the recommended 25 to 30 grams of fiber a day and have the greatest effect on your belly fat.

Time for a Change

I've addressed how sugar consumption has steadily climbed over 200 years. At the same time, consumption of complex carbs and fiber has declined greatly, with people typically eating fewer than 15 grams a day, which is about half the recommended amount. This combination of increased sugar and decreased fiber has had a drastic effect on the health of our country. That is why with the Carb Swap System, I'm suggesting a nationwide shift in common consumption patterns—this dramatic shift will truly transform health.

Start Today

With the Belly Fat Cure, you'll regain control of your confidence, your energy, and the most important part of your life: your health. The brand-new vitality you feel will empower you in every area—you'll reacquaint yourself with a level of confidence and security that will even carry over into your bedroom. Plus, you'll achieve a level of health that will ensure you end fatigue forever. You'll show your kids and loved ones how amazing living a healthy life can look and feel. Additionally, your risk of premature death will be significantly decreased, as will the threat of several diseases, including type 2 diabetes, heart disease, inflammation, and certain cancers. And, of course, you'll lose up to four to nine pounds of belly fat a week. Let's get started right now!

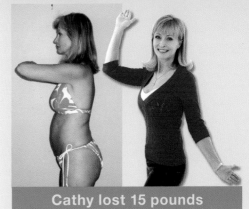

Cathy lost 15 pounds

Age: 54
Height: 5'6"
Pounds Lost: 15
Belly Inches Lost: 4

"I used to gain weight in my butt and thighs, but this time it was going right to my belly—and I knew that being an 'apple' was far more dangerous, health-wise, than being a 'pear.' I'm at the age where if I don't pay attention, I could easily lose control of my health; I intend to be active and on this earth for a long, long time. This plan is easy to follow, extremely effective, and a way of eating that I can truly live with. I don't have to decide to cheat or not—everything I want I can have, including wine!"

BEST TIP FOR SUCCESS:

"Use a food diary—it's a great tool to monitor progress, record history, and show what does and doesn't work."

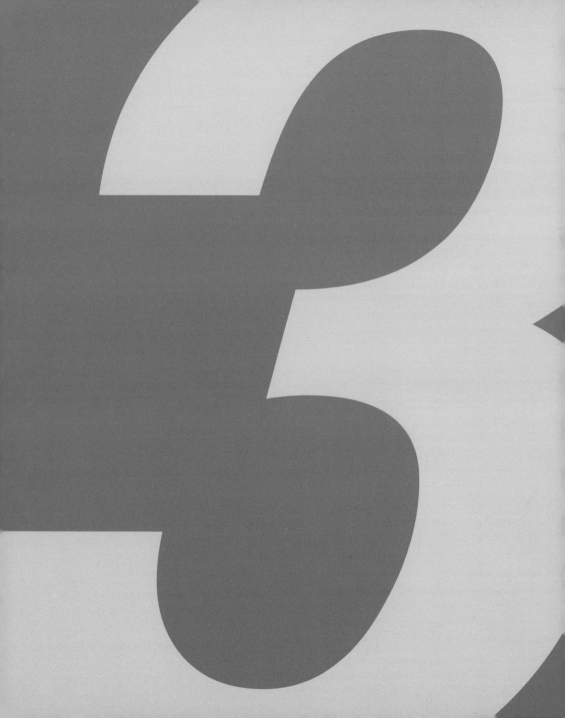

3 The One-Week Challenge and Beyond

I have created five different one-week meal plans to allow you to pick a menu that best fits your tastes and lifestyle. These five menus—Carb Lover, Meat Madness, Chicken & Seafood, Quick & Easy, and Sweet Bites—make losing four pounds a week super simple. I know you're going to love them. No thinking or guessing required; just follow any meal plan presented on the following pages. You can stick to a menu exactly as it's outlined for the entire week, or you can do one day's menu and on the next day switch to a new menu.

If you want to model my own "No-Excuses Day," follow the menu for what I eat almost every day, and you can consider it a basic blueprint for the Belly Fat Cure (check out pages 321–323 for gluten-free and vegetarian- and vegan-friendly No-Excuses Days). Feel free to use this on any day you want. As you can see, it's extremely easy:

1. Breakfast = three whole eggs, sunny-side up, and two pieces of toast with butter
2. Snack = a small handful of walnuts
3. Lunch = tuna salad on one piece of pita bread
4. Snack = one cup of cottage cheese sprinkled with an approved sweetener (page 267)
5. Dinner = grilled chicken or steak with sautéed veggies and a half cup of brown rice

Also, I make sure to drink eight to ten glasses of water a day and usually one Zevia soda. And when I get a sweet craving, I chew Spry gum. It's the perfect day!

Tracking Your Meals

On page 36 you'll find a planner on which you can track your meals. Make sure to make four copies of this planner, or join **TheBellyFatCure.com** free e-mail club to get access to a PDF copy that can be printed. Although the calculations on the challenge menus have been done for you, I urge you to use your tracker to gain a solid understanding of how the program works. Plus, I recommend using the daily mantra—"Instant health is my divine right, and I claim it now"—because it will help empower you emotionally. I start every day in this way, and I suggest that you do so as well in order to get that critical edge.

ONE-WEEK MENU: **CARB LOVER**

Satisfy your carb cravings without sabotaging your health. My team and I have developed delicious recipes that will allow you to lose weight while enjoying your favorite comfort foods, such as **Heavenly Berry Pancakes, Savory Pepperoni Pizza,** and **Creamy Chicken Alfredo Pasta.** Far from a diet, this is a lifestyle that incorporates all of the foods you love to eat.

	DAY 1	DAY 2	DAY 3	DAY 4	DAY 5
BREAKFAST	**Indulgent Cream-Cheese Toast** S/C Value = 3/2 page 79	**Parker's Old-Fashioned Pancakes** S/C Value = 0/2 page 43	**Berry Sweet Cereal** S/C Value = 3/2 page 75	**Heavenly Berry Pancakes** S/C Value = 2/2 page 47	**Sweet Apricot Oatmeal** S/C Value = 1/2 page 67
SNACK	**String Cheese** S/C Value = 0/0	**Hard-Boiled Egg** S/C Value = 0/0	**Walnuts (10)** S/C Value = 1/0	**Apricot (1 med.)** S/C Value = 3/0	**Almonds (10)** S/C Value = 1/0
LUNCH	**Superb Greek Pizza** S/C Value = 5/2 page 121	**Succulent Shrimp & Pesto Pasta** S/C Value = 5/2 page 143	**Savory Pepperoni Pizza** S/C Value = 4/2 page 103	**Super Tangy Chicken Wrap** S/C Value = 4/2 page 187	**Cheesy Enchiladas** S/C Value = 3/2 page 201
SNACK	**Jay Robb Protein Drink** S/C Value = 0/0	**Cottage Cheese (¼ cup)** S/C Value = 0/0	**Pecans (1 oz.)** S/C Value = 1/0	**1 Plain Rice Cake w/Cream Cheese** S/C Value = 0/0	**Dry-Roasted Pumpkin Seeds (¼ cup)** S/C Value = 0/0
DINNER	**Tuscan Basil Penne** S/C Value = 4/2 page 131	**Rich and Meaty Pasta Bake** S/C Value = 1/2 page 133	**Spicy Sausage Pasta** S/C Value = 2/2 page 127	**Extraordinary Mac 'n' Cheese** S/C Value = 2/2 page 139	**Creamy Chicken Alfredo Pasta** S/C Value = 4/2 page 137

DAY 6	DAY 7
Sweet Surprise Pancakes S/C Value = 0/2 page 45	**Blueberry Velvet Muffin** S/C Value = 0/2 page 81
Celery w/Cream Cheese S/C Value = 0/0	**Turkey & Cheese Roll** S/C Value = 0/0
Very Veggie Pizza S/C Value = 2/2 page 115	**Seasoned Chicken Burrito** S/C Value = 3/2 page 205
Brazil Nuts (6) S/C Value = 1/0	**Jay Robb Protein Drink** S/C Value = 0/0
Delightful Penne Pasta S/C Value = 3/2 page 125	**Ravioli Florentine** S/C Value = 2/2 page 135

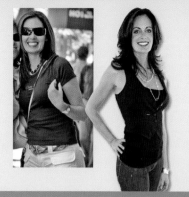

Heather lost 10 pounds

Age: 40
Height: 5'10"
Pounds Lost: 10
Belly Inches Lost: 3

"No matter how much I ran before, I could not lose that last five to seven pounds. I love to eat—I drink wine and have a lifestyle that's definitely about food, and I couldn't give that up. I've had friends in the past who have done Atkins and Jenny Craig, and they never stuck with it because they couldn't eat the foods they want to eat. On this plan, you can eat those foods all the time—and still see results. Once I received the information about where sugar was hiding (in things like milk!), the last bit of weight just came off. I am now down 10 pounds and feel better than I have in years."

BEST TIP FOR SUCCESS:

"Enjoy lattes with half-and-half—extra creamy and delicious!"

ONE-WEEK MENU: **MEAT MADNESS**

If you love steak, bacon, sausage, and ribs, then this is the menu for you! With incredible offerings such as **Rustic Steak & Cheese Panini, Wild-West Bacon Burger, Bold Pork Spareribs,** and **Gourmet Grilled Steak,** this menu is sure to satisfy even the heartiest of appetites.

	DAY 1	DAY 2	DAY 3	DAY 4	DAY 5
BREAKFAST	**First-Class French Toast** S/C Value = 4/2 page 51	**Sweet Surprise Pancakes** S/C Value = 0/2 page 45	**Super Cheesy Ham Omelette** S/C Value = 3/2 page 59	**Zesty Quiche Lorraine** S/C Value = 5/1 page 63	**Savory Breakfast Sandwich** S/C Value = 3/2 page 65
SNACK	**String Cheese** S/C Value = 0/0	**Hard-Boiled Egg** S/C Value = 0/0	**Walnuts (10)** S/C Value = 1/0	**String Cheese** S/C Value = 0/0	**Almonds (10)** S/C Value = 1/0
LUNCH	**Crispy Bacon Pizza** S/C Value = 3/2 page 105	**Simple Swiss & Mushroom Burger** S/C Value = 1/2 page 147	**Old-School BLT** S/C Value = 1/2 page 167	**Mouthwatering Meaty Pizza** S/C Value = 2/2 page 111	**Beef & Cheddar Sandwich** S/C Value = 2/2 page 171
SNACK	**Jay Robb Protein Drink** S/C Value = 0/0	**Cottage Cheese (¼ cup)** S/C Value = 0/0	**Pecans (10)** S/C Value = 1/0	**Blueberries (¼ cup)** S/C Value = 4/1	**Dry-Roasted Pumpkin Seeds (¼ cup)** S/C Value = 0/0
DINNER	**Sumptuous Pork Stir-Fry** S/C Value = 4/2 page 229	**Jorge's Carne Asada Tacos** S/C Value = 4/2 page 193	**Bountiful Steak Fajitas** S/C Value = 2/2 page 219	**Bold Pork Spareribs** S/C Value = 3/2 page 227	**Wild-West Bacon Burger** S/C Value = 2/2 page 151

DAY 6	DAY 7
Hearty Meat Scramble S/C Value = 2/2 **page 53**	**Perky Blended Coffee Shake** S/C Value = 0/1 **page 91**
Celery w/Cream Cheese S/C Value = 0/0	**Turkey & Cheese Roll** S/C Value = 0/0
Plentiful Italian Sub S/C Value = 4/2 **page 179**	**Rustic Steak & Cheese Panini** S/C Value = 1/2 **page 183**
Brazil Nuts (6) S/C Value = 1/0	**Blackberries (½ cup)** S/C Value = 4/1
Home-Style Meat Loaf S/C Value = 3/2 **page 223**	**Gourmet Grilled Steak** S/C Value = 3/2 **page 217**

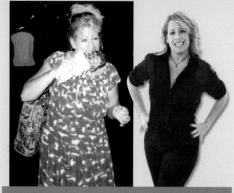

Kelly lost 17 pounds

Age: 41
Height: 5'4"
Pounds Lost: 17
Belly Inches Lost: 4.5

"I work in a doctor's office, and we have treats daily—like cookies, candies, and pastries—and I just became accustomed to eating this stuff all day long. With Jorge's plan, I've learned to prepare and really take care of myself. I've lost 17 pounds and feel better than ever. I have a ten-year-old daughter (my copilot) who is also learning about sugars, and she's helping me while helping herself. This program has changed my life; I've found something that truly works for me because it fits my lifestyle perfectly and can be done without struggle."

BEST TIP FOR SUCCESS:

"Persistence—just stick with it,
and the results will be
worth it!"

ONE-WEEK MENU: **CHICKEN & SEAFOOD**

Seafood and chicken are the mainstays of this menu, but we've added a few favorite turkey dishes as well. You'll be delighted by choices such as **Succulent Shrimp & Pesto Pasta, Pan-Seared Halibut,** and the **Ultimate Turkey Burger.** The breakfasts on this menu are also on the lighter side, including the **Lovely Layered Parfait** and the **Perky Blended Coffee Shake.**

	DAY 1	DAY 2	DAY 3	DAY 4	DAY 5
BREAKFAST	**Luscious Lox Bagel** S/C Value = 3/2 page 77	**Magical Mocha Blend** S/C Value = 0/1 page 95	**Savory Breakfast Sandwich** S/C Value = 3/2 page 65	**Go Nutty Shake** S/C Value = 1/2 page 87	**Lovely Layered Parfait** S/C Value = 5/2 page 69
SNACK	**String Cheese** S/C Value = 0/0	**Hard-Boiled Egg** S/C Value = 0/0	**Walnuts (10)** S/C Value = 1/0	**Nectarine (1 med.)** S/C Value = 5/1	**Almonds (10)** S/C Value = 1/0
LUNCH	**Tasty Margherita Pizza** S/C Value = 3/2 page 113	**Smokey Turkey Sandwich** S/C Value = 0/2 page 163	**Ultimate Turkey Burger** S/C Value = 1/2 page 161	**Robust BBQ Chicken Pizza** S/C Value = 2/2 page 107	**Tempting Tuna Sandwich** S/C Value = 1/2 page 175
SNACK	**Jay Robb Protein Drink** S/C Value = 0/0	**Blueberries (¼ cup)** S/C Value = 4/1	**Pecans (10)** S/C Value = 1/0	**String Cheese** S/C Value = 0/0	**Dry-Roasted Pumpkin Seeds (¼ cup)** S/C Value = 0/0
DINNER	**Ginger Grilled Shrimp** S/C Value = 2/2 page 241	**Succulent Shrimp & Pesto Pasta** S/C Value = 5/2 page 143	**Chipotle Chicken Tacos** S/C Value = 4/2 page 189	**Bacon & Feta Chicken Salad** S/C Value = 4/1 page 251	**Simple Shrimp Tacos** S/C Value = 5/2 page 197

DAY 6	DAY 7
Mediterranean Omelette S/C Value = 4/2 **page 61**	**Sweet Apricot Oatmeal** S/C Value = 1/2 **page 67**
Celery w/Cream Cheese S/C Value = 0/0	**Turkey & Cheese Roll** S/C Value = 0/0
Crispy Chicken Panini S/C Value = 3/2 **page 181**	**Classic Chicken Burger** S/C Value = 0/2 **page 155**
Brazil Nuts (6) S/C Value = 1/0	**Ruffles Original Potato Chips (1 oz.)** S/C Value = 0/1
Pan-Seared Halibut S/C Value = 1/2 **page 231**	**Owen's Finger-Lickin' Chicken Strips** S/C Value = 2/1 **page 209**

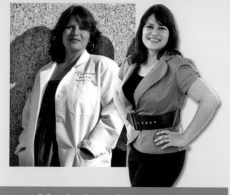

Maria lost 30 pounds

Age: 39
Height: 5'1"
Pounds Lost: 30
Belly Inches Lost: 6

"The Belly Fat Cure was my 'Aha!' moment. The program made me aware of a very important truth: I ate an excessive amount of sugar. Before, I was unaware that I had an unhealthy diet. I blamed my obesity on my genes, stress, and bad luck. I used to feel sluggish and tired every morning and evening. Now I'm eating healthier than ever before in my life, and I am much more confident in myself and feel good about my body. I feel younger, energized, and empowered. I feel inspired every day, and I have a new perspective on life!"

BEST TIP FOR SUCCESS:

"Keep a journal.
Be a meticulous accountant
of everything you eat.
This helped make me aware
of what I was eating."

ONE-WEEK MENU: **QUICK & EASY**

On the go? No time to cook? Then this is the perfect menu for you. With a mixture of microwavable frozen meals, fast food, and simple homemade options, you can stay on the plan with very little effort. Start your day off with a **Starbucks Bacon, Gouda, Cheese & Egg Frittata on an Artisan Roll** or some of my own **Berry Sweet Cereal,** then pop a **Lean Cuisine Shrimp Alfredo** in the microwave for lunch. Drive through Burger King on your way home, and end your day with a **Flame-Broiled Double Stacker.** It doesn't get any easier than this!

	DAY 1	DAY 2	DAY 3	DAY 4	DAY 5
BREAKFAST	**Starbucks Bacon, Gouda, Cheese & Egg Frittata on an Artisan Roll; with Coffee & Cream** S/C Value = 1/2	**Chocolate Lovers' Shake** S/C Value = 0/1 page 83	**Smooth Caramel Truffle Drink** S/C Value = 0/1 page 99	**Silky Vanilla Drink** S/C Value = 0/1 page 93	**Doctor's CarbRite Diet Bar (any flavor), with Coffee** S/C Value = 0/2 page 262
SNACK	**String Cheese** S/C Value = 0/0	**Hard-Boiled Egg** S/C Value = 0/0	**Walnuts (10)** S/C Value = 1/0	**Nectarine (1 med.)** S/C Value = 5/1	**Almonds (10)** S/C Value = 1/0
LUNCH	**2 Taco Bell Crunchy Taco Supreme Tacos, with Unsweetened Iced Tea** S/C Value = 4/2	**Lean Cuisine Alfredo Pasta with Chicken & Broccoli, with SoBe Black & Blue Berry Lifewater** S/C Value = 5/2	**Starbucks Rosemary Ham and Swiss Sandwich, with Ethos Water** S/C Value = 2/2	**Lean Cuisine Grilled Chicken Caesar, with Dasani Water** S/C Value = 2/2	**Starbucks Chop Chop Pasta Salad, with San Pellegrino Water** S/C Value = 2/2
SNACK	**Jay Robb Protein Drink** S/C Value = 0/0	**Blueberries (¼ cup)** S/C Value = 4/1	**Cheez-Its (27)** S/C Value = 0/1	**Blackberries (½ cup)** S/C Value = 4/1	**Celery w/Cream Cheese** S/C Value = 0/0
DINNER	**KFC Grilled Chicken Breast, Mashed Potatoes, Gravy, and Green Beans; with Aquafina Water** S/C Value = 1/2	**Lean Cuisine Chicken Carbonara, with Dasani Lime Essence Flavored Water** S/C Value = 3/2	**Carl's Jr./ Hardee's Spicy Chicken Sandwich** S/C Value = 3/2	**KFC Grilled Chicken Wings w/Mac & Cheese** S/C Value = 4/1	**Lean Cuisine Swedish Meatballs, with Perrier Water** S/C Value = 4/2

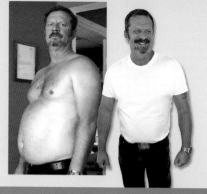

DAY 6	DAY 7
Energize Me Green Tea S/C Value = 1/1 **page 97**	**Berry Sweet Cereal** S/C Value = 3/2 **page 75**
Tortilla Chips (10) & Salsa (2 Tbsp.) S/C Value =0/1	**Turkey & Cheese Roll** S/C Value = 0/0
Lean Cuisine Shrimp Alfredo with SoBe Acai Fruit Punch Lifewater S/C Value = 5/2	**Starbucks Turkey & Swiss Sandwich, with Unsweetened Iced Tea** S/C Value = 5/2
Brazil Nuts (6) S/C Value = 0/0	**Ruffles Original Potato Chips (1 oz.)** S/C Value = 0/1
Carl's Jr./ Hardee's Jumbo Chili Dog S/C Value = 4/2	**Lean Cuisine Steak Tips Portabello, with SoBe Mango Melon Lifewater** S/C Value = 3/1

Russ lost 13 pounds

Age: 51
Height: 5'11"
Pounds Lost: 13
Belly Inches Lost: 5.5

"I used to have several health issues associated with being overweight, but paramount was my low self-esteem. I was borrowing clothes because I couldn't wear my own, and I refused to buy new ones because that meant I was resolved to being fat. Within a very short period of time, I was able to get back into my clothes and get back to living my life and being social. I used to have abdominal pain because my organs were pressing against one another, and lower back pain because of my belly fat—that's all gone now. I have a healthier lifestyle and a more pleasant outlook on life."

BEST TIP FOR SUCCESS:

"Keep the recommended snacks around to help avoid the 'run to the 7-Eleven for a treat' trips."

ONE-WEEK MENU: **SWEET BITES**

If you have a sweet tooth, this is definitely the menu for you. Here, salads and lighter lunches are featured to leave room for those sweet treats you just can't do without. You'll find **Gooey Caramel Pancakes; Sweet Hawaiian Pizza; Summer Spinach Salad;** and, of course, plenty of chocolate and ice cream!

	DAY 1	DAY 2	DAY 3	DAY 4	DAY 5
BREAKFAST	**Sweet Surprise Pancakes** S/C Value = 0/2 page 45	**Chocolate Lovers' Shake** S/C Value = 0/1 page 83	**Blueberry Velvet Muffins** S/C Value = 0/2 page 81	**Heavenly Berry Pancakes** S/C Value = 2/2 page 47	**Sweet Strawberry Smoothie** S/C Value = 3/2 page 85
LUNCH	**Quattro Formaggio Pizza** S/C Value = 2/2 page 109	**Chicken Caesar Salad Wrap** S/C Value = 2/2 page 185	**Pecan Delight Chopped Salad** S/C Value = 3/1 page 261	**Sweet Hawaiian Pizza** S/C Value = 5/2 page 119	**Ham & Cheese Sandwich** S/C Value = 2/2 page 169
SNACK	**Pecans** S/C Value = 1/0	**String Cheese** S/C Value = 0/0	**Hard-Boiled Egg** S/C Value = 0/0	**Turkey & Cheese Roll** S/C Value = 0/0	**Walnuts (10)** S/C Value = 1/0
DINNER	**Lovely Cobb Salad** S/C Value = 3/1 page 249	**Gourmet Grilled Steak** S/C Value = 3/2 page 217	**Seaside Tacos** S/C Value = 5/2 page 191	**Owen's Finger-Lickin' Chicken Strips** S/C Value = 2/1 page 209	**Bacon & Feta Chicken Salad** S/C Value = 4/1 page 251
TREAT	**½ cup Clemmy's Chocolate Ice Cream** S/C Value = 0/1	**½ cup Clemmy's Vanilla Bean Ice Cream** S/C Value = 0/1	**12 pieces Green & Black's Dark 85% Chocolate** S/C Value = 5/1	**½ cup Clemmy's Chocolate Ice Cream** S/C Value = 0/1	**½ cup Clemmy's Vanilla Bean Ice Cream** S/C Value = 0/1

DAY 6	DAY 7
Gooey Caramel Pancakes S/C Value = 1/2 **page 49**	**Frosty Berry Shake** S/C Value = 2/2 **page 89**
Crunchy Sesame Chicken Salad S/C Value = 3/1 **page 253**	**Summer Spinach Salad** S/C Value = 0/1 **page 257**
Celery w/Cream Cheese S/C Value = 0/0	**Hard-Boiled Egg** S/C Value = 0/0
Pizza Blanca S/C Value = 2/2 **page 117**	**The Best Holiday Dinner** S/C Value = 3/2 **page 211**
12 pieces Green & Black's Dark 85% Chocolate S/C Value = 5/1	**½ cup Clemmy's Vanilla Bean Ice Cream** S/C Value = 0/1

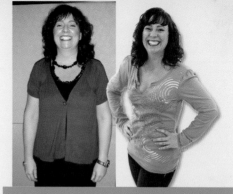

Tina lost 15 pounds

Age: 39
Height: 5'2"
Pounds Lost: 15
Belly Inches Lost: 7

"After a horrible divorce, I was constantly tired, yet I couldn't sleep. I was overweight and had tried many programs that always led to more weight gain later. I had back and joint pain . . . in short, I needed a miracle, and I found it in this plan. I quickly had more energy, I was sleeping through the night, my pain began to subside, and somehow I was eating more than ever and losing weight and inches. The best part is that I was able to eat all the things I love: eggs, bacon, ice cream, chocolate, and wine. I love this program; it really is a lifestyle!"

BEST TIP FOR SUCCESS:

"Make dinners
for at least five nights
on Sunday."

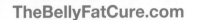

TheBellyFatCure.com

STEP 1: GET CONTROL

Upon waking, repeat this mantra out loud ten times to gain control of your day:

Instant health is my divine right, and I claim it now.

STEP 2: EAT USING S/C VALUE

INSTRUCTIONS: Cross off one sugar per gram consumed, and cross off one carbohydrate per serving consumed.

Sugar (15 Grams) ○ ○ ○ ○ ○ ○ ○ ○ ○ ○ ○ ○ ○ ○ ○

Carbs* (6 Servings) ○ ○ ○ ○ ○ ○

*Note: 1 serving of Carbs is 5 to 20 grams

TheBellyFatCure.com

STEP 1: GET CONTROL

Upon waking, repeat this mantra out loud ten times to gain control of your day:

Instant health is my divine right, and I claim it now.

STEP 2: EAT USING S/C VALUE

INSTRUCTIONS: Cross off one sugar per gram consumed, and cross off one carbohydrate per serving consumed.

Sugar (15 Grams) ○ ○ ○ ○ ○ ○ ○ ○ ○ ○ ○ ○ ○ ○ ○

Carbs* (6 Servings) ○ ○ ○ ○ ○ ○

*Note: 1 serving of Carbs is 5 to 20 grams

Planner Instructions:

As I shared with you in Chapter 2, the S/C Value is the secret code that will unlock the combination to the Belly Fat Cure. Your daily S/C Value is 15/6 (no more than 15 grams of sugar and 6 servings of carbs). Simply cross off one sugar box for every gram of sugar consumed and one carbohydrate box for each serving of carbs consumed.

Carbohydrate servings are counted as follows:

- 0 to 4 carbohydrate grams = not counted
- 5 to 20 carbohydrate grams = 1 serving
- 21 to 40 carbohydrate grams = 2 servings
- 41 to 60 carbohydrate grams = 3 servings

But you won't have to worry about converting carb grams to servings if you're following the one-week challenge menus. For each item, you'll find a page number listed where you'll see the S/C Value for each meal. For example, the Jumbo Shrimp Fajitas on page 245 show an S/C Value of 5/2. For this meal, you'd cross off five sugar boxes and two carbohydrate-serving boxes.

Beyond the One-Week Challenge

After your one-week challenge, you'll have just two questions:

1. *How do I lose more?* and
2. *How do I maintain my results?*

What follows are the answers to these two important questions.

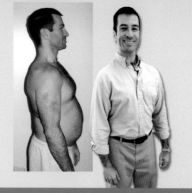

Ken lost 10 pounds

Age: 46
Height: 5'8"
Pounds Lost: 10
Belly Inches Lost: 4

"A big belly has interfered in just about every area of my life: at work, at home, at the beach, and at the gym. It's also made it painful for me to stretch and do the exercises I love. I used to avoid getting my picture taken because my self-esteem was so low. I've been dieting forever, trying to get rid of this belly—the fat affects every aspect of my life. After just two weeks on the Belly Fat Cure, I started getting compliments and feeling my confidence come back. I even went up to the attic to get my skinny pants, and I'm going to need new belts soon—this is after just two weeks! My belly is disappearing!"

BEST TIP FOR SUCCESS:

"Realize that getting rid of your belly will truly change your life; make the commitment to yourself to stick with it."

How to Lose More

Simply stick to the meals featured in the one-week challenge for as long as you like. Ideally, you'll try all five of our menus for some great variety. You're going to love them all, including the Quick & Easy menu that's super fast and perfect for when you're traveling or short on time! Of course you can dig in to the more than 100 Carb Swap recipes in Chapter 4 and simply pick three a day to enjoy. It's truly that easy! (And if you do want to lose more, it's a good idea to read the FAQs at the end of the book for more vital answers to the program.)

If you ever hit a plateau, I recommend that you return to the tracker to make sure that you're sticking to the 15/6 formula each day. Tracking what you eat every day will help keep you accountable and ensure that you're eating exactly what you need to maximize belly fat loss. Plus, really pay attention to how much fiber you're getting on a daily basis—aim for 25 to 30 grams and you'll be amazed by how quickly your false belly fat disappears. I also recommend referring back to the chart on page 4; if you're near your goal weight, your weight loss will naturally slow down a bit.

Be sure to take advantage of all of the other tools included in this book. Turn to Chapter 6 for the food list that has hundreds of items listed with their S/C Value. Use this with your daily eating to help you make smarter choices and live the Belly Fat Cure lifestyle. And in Chapter 5, you'll find a grocery-products list with more than 800 items with their S/C Value (including pictures). You can refer back to this list whenever you have questions about a food's sugar and carb content, and I recommend that you become very familiar with it because it will be one of your best resources on this plan.

How to Maintain Your Results

If you want to maintain your results, it's easy—make the plan a lifestyle! Just continue to follow my recommended daily S/C Value of 15/6. It's how I live my own life.

My clients often ask me if they really need to continue to minimize fruit consumption to be successful on this program in the long run. Well, until they've reached their goal weight or a healthy waist circumference, I strongly suggest that they temporarily limit it by choosing low-sugar fruits such as blueberries and blackberries. The naturally occurring sugar found in fruits (fructose) is still sugar, and it has the same impact on belly fat—it helps promote it. The quickest way to get rid of that stubborn belly fat, and to make sure it stays off, is to adhere to my recommendation of consuming no more than 15 grams of sugar each day, regardless of the source.

While fruit does contain beneficial vitamins, minerals, and antioxidants, it isn't essential to eat it to receive the benefits. There are many great supplements that provide important vitamins like vitamin C. Also, look to vegetable sources as well: bell peppers, broccoli, and brussels sprouts all have more vitamin C than oranges do, for example. Once you've reached your goal weight, you may slowly incorporate up to two additional pieces of fruit back into your diet. Limit it to no more than two extra pieces per day, and do try to eat local, seasonal fruit in its complete, natural form (with the skin on) whenever possible.

Monitor the effect that the added fruit has on your body, and be your own judge of the proper amount for you. If you're an active person, chances are you'll be able to enjoy fruit without a negative impact. Just remember to avoid it in extremely high-sugar forms such as smoothies and juices.

Living the Belly Fat Cure lifestyle will absolutely give you optimal health, as well as the most attractive waistline you can have. You'll have an unstoppable immune system, endless energy, and a much lower risk for the most deadly diseases—there's no looking back!

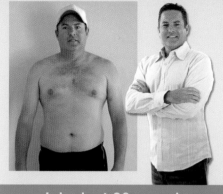

John lost 36 pounds

Age: 46
Height: 5'11"
Pounds Lost: 36
Belly Inches Lost: 10

"I'd been struggling with my weight for more than a decade. In the last seven years, both of my parents passed away from health issues at an earlier than expected age (from cancer and heart disease). Now, at the age of 46, my wife and I have a 15-year-old daughter and a 22-month-old son—I have to stay young and healthy for them! This program was like somebody turned on a light switch in my head . . . it all began to make sense. It has definitely been the easiest lifestyle change I've ever made. I'm so excited about the future."

BEST TIP FOR SUCCESS:

"Purchase a small cooler or lunch box and make sure you have ½ cup plastic containers and Baggies available to pack meals."

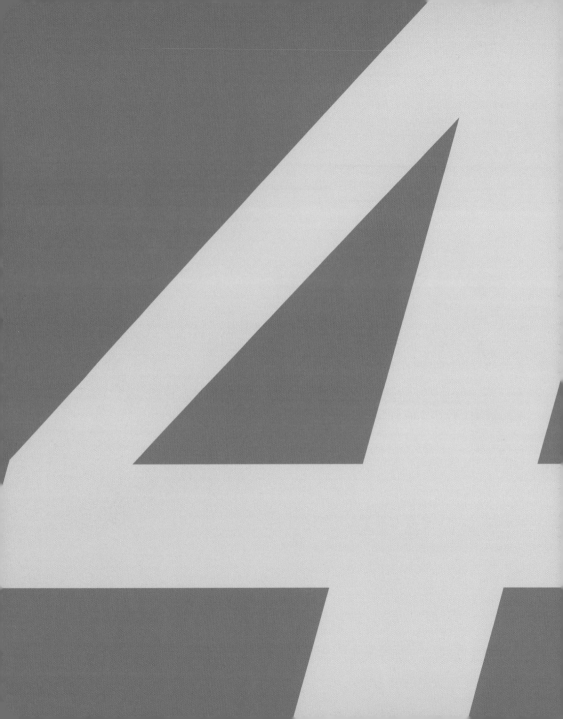

4 Carb Swap
Meals

In this chapter, you'll find more than 100 Belly Good Carb Swap meals. My goal in creating these recipes was to make sure that they were delicious, cost-effective, and quick to make. Yet all of these meals also have an S/C Value of 5/2 or less. As you know, with the Belly Fat Cure you get 15 grams of sugar and 6 carb servings per day, which means that you can mix and match any 3 of these meals every day and see amazing results. You'll also notice that every recipe has an example of a Belly Bad meal that will serve as a shocking comparison.

Note that almost all of these Belly Good meals serve 4—that's because they're so delicious, you'll want to serve them to your whole family or have quick leftovers to make your eating even simpler. You'll also notice that some of the meals say "season to taste"; you may season freely with salt, pepper, herbs, and/or your favorite sugar-free spices.

The exciting part about learning this new eating method will be discovering and trying new, delicious products. **If some of the brand names look unfamiliar to you, make sure to check page 262 for the Websites of these products.** If for some reason you're not able to easily obtain the products we suggest in the recipe, feel free to substitute with any low-sugar and/or whole-grain version you find locally. Also, don't be afraid to get creative with some of the recipes. For example, if you can't find the bread we recommend for the First-Class French Toast on page 51, use an everyday light bread instead and just eat 2 pieces instead of 4. Either way, you're gong to love eating my Belly Fat Cure–Approved Meals—they're delicious!

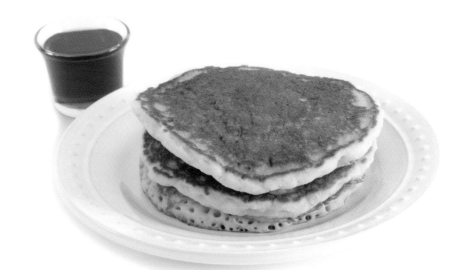

BELLY BAD

S/C Value = 42/6

BELLY GOOD

S/C Value = 0/2

Denny's Buttermilk Pancakes

Since syrup is typically made by dissolving sugar in water, it requires outrageous amounts of sugar to generate a small amount (see page 273 for a smarter syrup).

Buttermilk Pancakes Do-Over

Using soy flour instead of regular flour cuts the carb grams by more than half. I like the Arrowhead Mills brand, but any soy flour will do.

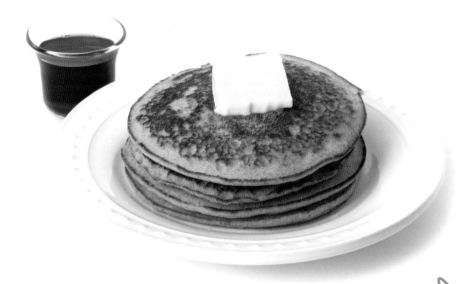

Parker's Old-Fashioned Pancakes

Serves 4

Pancakes:

2⅓ cups Arrowhead Mills Organic Soy Flour
2 Tbsp. plus ½ tsp. baking powder
1 tsp. xylitol
½ tsp. salt
4 eggs
1⅓ cups half-and-half
⅓ cup Almond Breeze Vanilla Unsweetened
   Almond Milk
⅔ cup water
5 Tbsp. melted butter, divided use

Other sides:

8 Tbsp. Joseph's Sugar Free Maple Syrup
4 Tbsp. butter

1. Sift together the flour, baking powder, xylitol, and salt into a large bowl; set aside. In a medium bowl, whisk together eggs, half-and-half, almond milk, and water until blended.

2. Make a well in the center of the dry ingredients. Pour wet ingredients into the well and stir until just combined. Blend in 4 Tbsp. of the melted butter.

3. Heat a large skillet over medium heat. Add the remaining Tbsp. of butter to the pan. Add about ⅓ cup of batter per pancake and cook until golden brown and bubbly. Flip over and cook about 45 seconds more. Repeat until the batter is gone.

4. Top each stack of pancakes with a Tbsp. of butter and serve with a side of syrup.

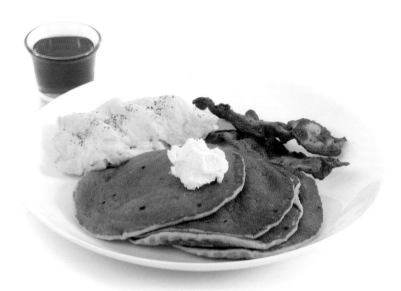

BELLY BAD

S/C Value = 202/18

BELLY GOOD

S/C Value = 0/2

Mimi's Café Banana Chocolate Chip Pancake Breakfast

This dish might not look overly sweet, but it's actually packed with 202 grams of sugar—the equivalent of almost 2 weeks' worth of sugar on the Belly Fat Cure.

Banana Chocolate Chip Pancake Do-Over:

I love to make this on Sundays for my sons, Parker and Owen. Make it and no one will ever know that it's healthy, too. Yummy!

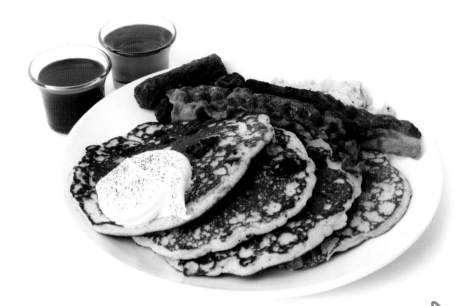

Sweet Surprise Pancakes

Serves 4

Pancakes:
Refer to page 43
¼ cup Hershey's Sugar Free Chocolate Chips

Chocolate sauce:
¼ cup Hershey's Sugar Free Chocolate Chips
¼ cup whipping cream

Whipped-cream topping:
¼ cup cold whipping cream
1 tsp. xylitol
1 pinch unsweetened cocoa powder

Other sides:
4 eggs
8 strips of bacon
8 sausage links
8 Tbsp. Joseph's Sugar Free Maple Syrup

1. For the pancakes: Follow the recipe from page 43, stirring the chocolate chips into the batter at the same time as the melted butter.

2. For the chocolate sauce: In a small saucepan over low heat, heat the rest of the chocolate chips and the whipping cream, stirring constantly until the chocolate is melted and the sauce is smooth.

3. For the whipped cream: In a small mixing bowl, whip the cream with xylitol until soft peaks form.

4. For the eggs and meats: Cook as desired.

5. Top the pancakes with a dollop of whipped cream and a pinch of cocoa. Serve with a side of chocolate sauce and syrup, along with the eggs and meats.

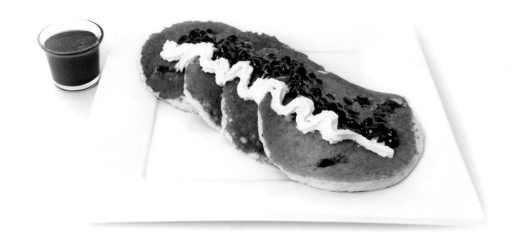

BELLY BAD

S/C Value = 46/7

IHOP Double Blueberry Pancakes

IHOP doesn't publish its nutritional information—kind of makes it hard to eat healthfully, doesn't it? My team and I used data from a popular nutrition site and verified it in-house.

BELLY GOOD

S/C Value = 2/2

Double Blueberry Pancakes Do-Over:

Blackberries and raspberries are two of my top recommendations for fruit; they are high in antioxidants that help prevent cancer and are low-sugar fruits.

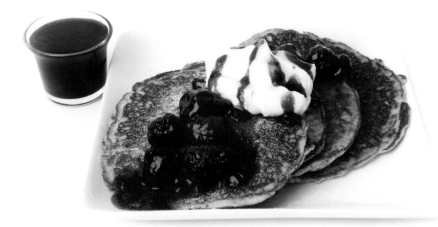

Heavenly Berry Pancakes

Serves 4

Pancakes:
Refer to page 43

Berry topping:
⅓ cup Nature's Hollow Sugar Free Mountain
   Berry Preserves
¼ cup water
½ cup blackberries
½ cup raspberries

Whipped-cream topping:
4 Tbsp. cold whipping cream
1 tsp. xylitol

Other sides:
8 Tbsp. Nature's Hollow Sugar Free
   Raspberry Syrup
1 tsp. xylitol

1. For the pancakes: Make pancakes from page 43.

2. For the berry topping: Heat the preserves, water, and berries in a saucepan over medium heat, stirring frequently, until the berries start to break down and the preserves have melted. Bring to a simmer; remove from heat and set aside.

3. For the whipped cream: In a separate bowl, whip cream with xylitol until peaks form.

4. Top pancakes with a dollop of whipped cream, then add the berry topping and sprinkle with xylitol. Serve with a side of syrup.

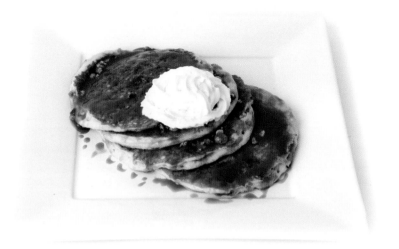

BELLY BAD

S/C Value = 53/7

IHOP Butterscotch Rocks Pancakes

Since IHOP doesn't make its nutritional information available to the public, my nutritional team broke down this meal and created an S/C Value for it.

BELLY GOOD

S/C Value = 1/2

Butterscotch Rocks Pancakes Do-Over:

It's hard to believe that you can enjoy these amazing-looking pancakes and eat just 1 gram of sugar and 2 carb servings.

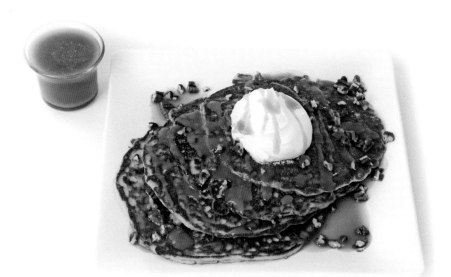

Gooey Caramel Pancakes

Serves 4

Pancakes:
Refer to page 43

Caramel sauce:
½ cup Seelect Teas' Organic Caramel Syrup
½ cup whipping cream at room temperature

Whipped-cream topping:
4 Tbsp. cold whipping cream
1 tsp. xylitol

Other sides:
4 Tbsp. chopped pecans

1. For the pancakes: Make pancakes from page 43.

2. For the caramel sauce: In a small bowl, combine the caramel syrup with whipping cream. Set aside.

3. For the whipped cream: In a separate bowl, whip the cold whipping cream with xylitol until peaks form.

4. Top pancakes with pecans, a dollop of whipped cream, and caramel sauce. Serve with a side of remaining caramel sauce if desired.

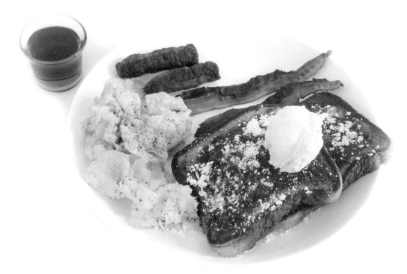

BELLY BAD

S/C Value = 42/6

BELLY GOOD

S/C Value = 4/2

Denny's French Toast Slam

Enjoy the protein sides from this dish—the eggs, sausage, and bacon—but skip the French toast if you want to lose belly fat and regain your health and energy.

French Toast Do-Over:

My team and I used bread from Ener-G Foods, which has the lowest carb value of any bread we found. Cinnamon also helps control blood sugar when consumed with carbs.

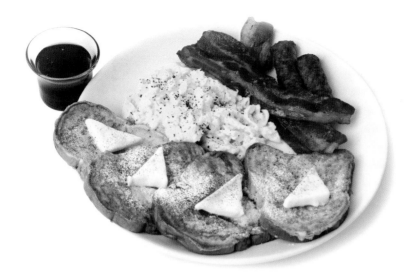

First-Class French Toast

Serves 4

French toast:
3 eggs
¾ cup half-and-half
1 tsp. cinnamon
¼ tsp. nutmeg
2 Tbsp. butter
16 slices Ener-G Foods Light Brown Rice Loaf

Other sides:
1 Tbsp. butter
8 whole eggs
8 strips of bacon
8 sausage links
2 packets stevia powder
½ cup Joseph's Sugar Free Maple Syrup

1. For the French toast: Melt butter in a large skillet or griddle. Whisk the eggs, half-and-half, cinnamon, and nutmeg in a medium-sized bowl. Dip slices of bread through the egg mixture, one at a time, turning once until bread is well coated. Add bread to the skillet and cook 3 minutes per side or until golden brown.

2. For the eggs and meats: Cook as desired.

3. Sprinkle the French toast with stevia and top with butter. Serve with the eggs and meats, as well as a side of syrup.

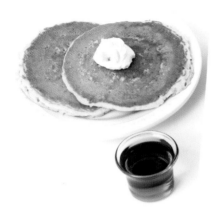

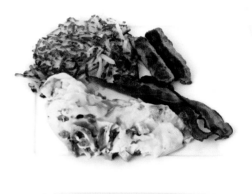

BELLY BAD

S/C Value = 40/6

BELLY GOOD

S/C Value = 2/2

Denny's Meat Lover's Scramble

This meal has almost
3 days' worth of sugar
on the Belly Fat Cure.
Plus, the carb count
of this meal will knock out
a whole day's worth
in one shot.

Meat Lover's Scramble Do-Over:

Enjoy saturated fats in
moderation; for example,
if you have this meal for
breakfast, balance out your
day with a salad for lunch
and a chicken- or veggie-
pasta dish for dinner.

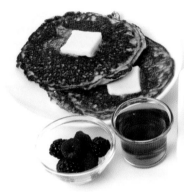
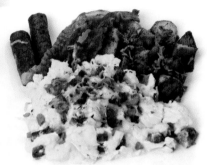

Hearty Meat Scramble

Serves 4

Scramble:
1 Tbsp. butter
¼ lb. breakfast sausage, crumbled and browned
3 strips of bacon, cooked and chopped
2 slices of ham, diced (approximately ⅓ cup)
12 whole eggs
¼ cup half-and-half
Salt and pepper to taste
½ cup shredded cheddar cheese
2 green onions, green parts only, thinly sliced

Other sides:
1 cup Simply Potatoes Red Potato Wedges
½ recipe Parker's Old-Fashioned Pancakes
    (refer to page 43; yields 8 pancakes)
8 Tbsp. Joseph's Sugar Free Maple Syrup
1 Tbsp. seasoning for potatoes
8 strips of bacon
8 sausage links
1 cup mixed berries (raspberries & blackberries)

1. For the scramble: Warm a skillet over medium heat; add butter until melted. Add cooked sausage, cooked bacon, and ham; sauté 2 minutes. Whisk the eggs with half-and-half and season with salt and pepper in a separate bowl. Add the egg mixture to the skillet; scramble until the eggs are cooked almost through. Add the cheese and cook until melted.

2. For the potatoes and meats: Cook as desired and season to taste.

3. For the pancakes: Make half of the recipe for Parker's Old-Fashioned Pancakes from page 43.

4. Garnish the scramble with chopped green onions. Serve with the meats and a side of potatoes, and with pancakes topped with butter and berries. Serve warm syrup on the side.

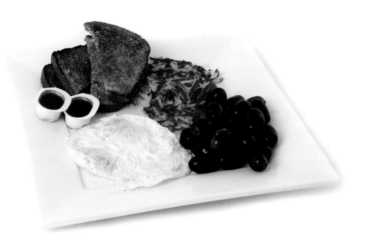

BELLY BAD

S/C Value = 30/5

BELLY GOOD

S/C Value = 4/2

Denny's Build Your Own Grand Slam

Jelly has about 12 grams of sugar in 1 Tbsp.; I recommend just butter on your toast when given the option in a restaurant. See page 273 for better jelly choices.

Grand Slam Do-Over:

When you eat eggs sunny-side up, you get more nutrients from yolks that are uncooked.

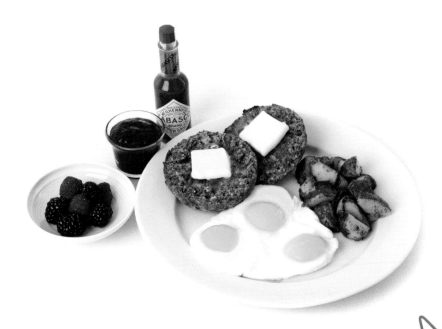

Sunny-Side Breakfast

Serves 4

Eggs:
3 Tbsp. butter, divided
12 eggs

Other sides:
1 cup Simply Potatoes Red Potato Wedges
½ cup mixed blackberries and raspberries
4 Rudi's Organic Bakery Whole Grain Wheat
    English Muffins
¼ cup Nature's Hollow Sugar Free Preserves
    (any flavor)
Tabasco Pepper Sauce to taste

1. For the eggs: Warm a nonstick skillet over medium heat; add butter until melted. Cooking three at a time, crack each egg separately into the pan; season to taste with salt and pepper. Fry for 1 to 2 minutes or until the whites are set, then remove the eggs from the pan with a non-metal spatula. Repeat with the remaining eggs.

2. For the potatoes: Cook according to package directions.

3. Serve the eggs and potatoes with a toasted and buttered English muffin; along with some mixed berries, preserves, and Tabasco.

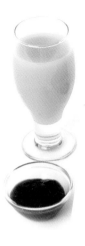
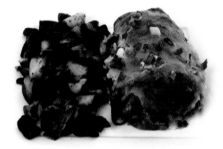

BELLY BAD

S/C Value = 42/8

Mimi's Café Chipotle Breakfast Burrito

It takes up to 4 oranges to make a glass of orange juice, which adds up to more than 20 grams of sugar. The same is true of all fruit juices.

BELLY GOOD

S/C Value = 2/2

Chipotle Breakfast Burrito Do-Over:

Instead of juice, try an Ultima Replenisher Orange drink—it is filled with tons of great vitamins and is sweetened with stevia, a natural sweetener.

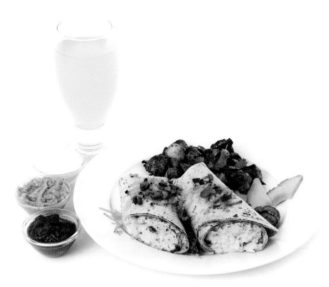

South of the Border Burrito

Serves 4

Burrito:

1 Tbsp. butter

8 whole eggs

¼ cup half-and-half

½ lb. breakfast sausage

½ cup Jack cheese, or packaged shredded Mexican blend

4 Tbsp. La Victoria Salsa Suprema Mild, drained well

4 Food for Life Ezekiel 4:9 Sprouted Grain Tortillas

¼ cup cilantro, chopped

Other sides:

1 cup Simply Potatoes Red Potato Wedges

1 avocado, mashed (leave 8 thin slices for garnish)

4 Tbsp. sour cream

4 jalapeños, charred

8 oz. water

1 packet Ultima Replenisher Orange drink

1. For the burrito: Melt the butter in a large skillet over medium heat. Crumble the sausage into the skillet, breaking it up with the back of a wooden spoon, and cook until browned. In a separate bowl, whisk the eggs with the half-and-half, and season to taste. Add the egg mixture to the pan and scramble; when the eggs are almost set, add the cheese. When the cheese has melted, add the drained salsa, stirring well to combine.

2. Warm the tortillas over a gas flame or in a pan, then fill with ¼ of the egg mixture; top with cilantro. Fold up the bottom part of tortilla, then roll each side over.

3. For the potatoes: Cook according to package directions.

4. Cut each burrito in half; garnish with the charred jalapeño, cheese, and sliced avocado. Serve with the potatoes, along with a smashed avocado and sour cream on the side. Prepare the orange drink and pour into juice glasses.

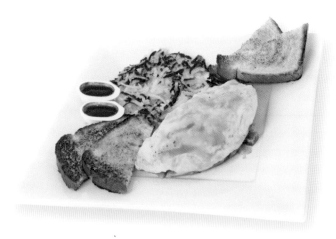

BELLY BAD

S/C Value = 18/4

Denny's Ham & Cheddar Omelette

Denny's white bread is made with processed white flour and doesn't have any of the beneficial whole grains that are recommended for getting rid of belly fat.

BELLY GOOD

S/C Value = 3/2

Ham & Cheddar Omelette Do-Over:

Cheese is one of my favorite foods because it is a good source of protein and tastes great. Plus, it has a 0/0 S/C Value.

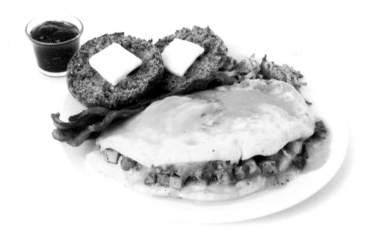

Super Cheesy Ham Omelette

Serves 1

Omelette:
3 eggs
2 Tbsp. half-and-half
Salt and pepper, to taste
Cooking spray
2 slices of ham, diced (approximately ⅓ cup)
¼ cup shredded cheddar cheese

Other sides:
1 Rudi's Organic Bakery Whole Grain Wheat
   English Muffin
1 Tbsp. butter
1 Tbsp. Nature's Hollow Sugar Free Raspberry
   Preserves
½ cup Cascadian Farm Hash Browns
2 strips of bacon, cooked

1. For the omelette: Whisk the eggs and half-and-half; season to taste. Heat a small nonstick pan over medium-low heat, and spray cooking spray liberally over the pan. Add the egg mixture and swirl to coat the pan; leave and let the eggs "set up." When the sides start to pull away, add ham and cheese to half of the pan. Fold one side over the other, creating a half moon, and remove from heat.

2. For the potatoes and bacon: Cook according to package directions.

3. Serve the omelette with bacon, hash browns, a buttered and toasted English muffin, and a side of preserves.

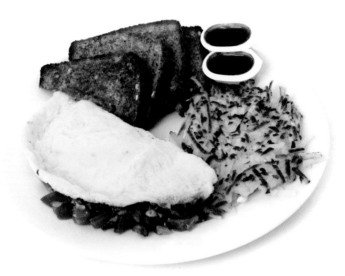

BELLY BAD

S/C Value = 24/4

Denny's Veggie-Cheese Omelette with Egg Beaters

You can enjoy a veggie omelette, but you just have to make smart choices about the vegetables you use.

BELLY GOOD

S/C Value = 4/2

Veggie-Cheese Omelette Do-Over:

Spinach is a good source of fiber and several important vitamins and minerals, and it's an excellent source of vitamin K, which is critical for bone health.

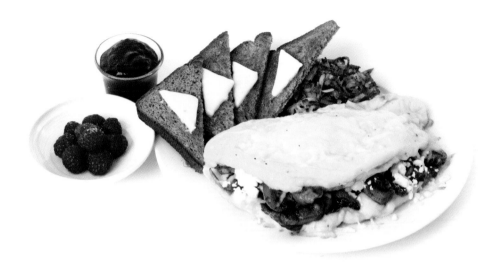

Mediterranean Omelette

Serves 1

Omelette:
3 eggs
2 Tbsp. half-and-half
Salt, pepper, and Lawry's Lemon Pepper
    Seasoning; to taste
1 Tbsp. butter
1 garlic clove, minced
2 button mushrooms, chopped
2 Tbsp. green onions, chopped
¼ cup spinach
2 Tbsp. feta cheese
2 basil leaves, chopped
Cooking spray

Other sides:
2 slices Food for Life Ezekiel 4:9 Sprouted 100%
    Whole Grain Bread
2 pats of butter
½ cup Cascadian Farm Hash Browns
¼ cup raspberries
1 Tbsp. Nature's Hollow Sugar Free Preserves

1. For the omelette: Whisk eggs with the half-and-half, salt, pepper, and Lawry's seasoning; set aside. Heat a small nonstick skillet over medium-low heat; add butter. When the butter has melted, sauté the vegetables for about 3 minutes; remove from pan and set aside. Wipe out the pan and spray cooking spray lightly over the pan; add the egg mixture and swirl around. Cook eggs undisturbed until set. Add the sautéed vegetables, feta, and chopped basil to half of the pan. Fold one side of the omelette over the other to form a half moon. Remove from heat, and slide the omelette onto your plate.

2. For the hash browns: Cook according to package directions.

3. Serve the omelette with toast, hash browns, and a side of berries and preserves.

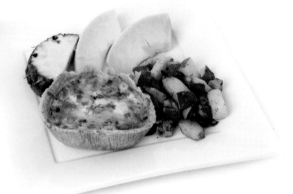
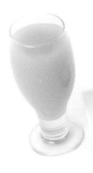

BELLY BAD

S/C Value = 24/4

Mimi's Café Quiche Lorraine with Bacon and Swiss Cheese

The quiche alone has 12 grams of sugar. Pair it with high-sugar fruits like pineapple and honeydew melon, and you get a belly fat–promoting meal—even before getting to the juice.

BELLY GOOD

S/C Value = 5/1

Quiche Lorraine Do-Over:

Enjoy this meal with a cup of coffee, which is actually one of the top sources of antioxidants in the American diet. See page 267 for sweetener options.

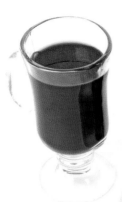
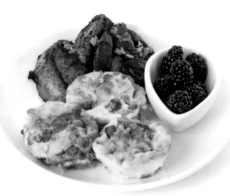

Zesty Quiche Lorraine

Serves 4

Quiche:

6 whole eggs

4 Tbsp. half-and-half

Tabasco Pepper Sauce or your favorite hot sauce, to taste

Salt and pepper, to taste

Cooking spray

¼ cup grated Swiss cheese

3 green onions, green parts only, thinly sliced

8 strips of bacon cooked and chopped (or ½ cup either ham or pancetta, chopped)

Other sides:

2 cups Simply Potatoes Rosemary & Garlic Red Potato Wedges

1 cup blackberries

1 cup of coffee per person

1. For the quiche: Preheat oven to 350° F. Whisk the eggs, half-and-half, and Tabasco until combined. Add the cheese and onion; season to taste with salt and pepper. Coat a 12-muffin tin with cooking spray. Divide the meat into each muffin cup and top with the egg mixture. Bake for approximately 15–18 minutes or until a knife inserted in the middle of the quiche comes out clean. Let stand 5 minutes and serve.

2. For the potatoes: Prepare according to package directions.

3. Serve 3 quiches per person with equal amounts of potatoes and fruit, and 1 cup of coffee.

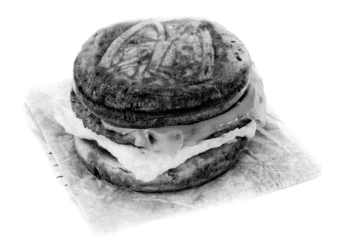

BELLY BAD

S/C Value = 15/3

McDonald's Sausage McGriddles

The meat, cheese, and egg here aren't bad, but the pancakes-as-bread feature give this little sandwich 15 grams of sugar—that's a whole day's worth on the Belly Fat Cure.

BELLY GOOD

S/C Value = 3/2

Sausage McGriddles Do-Over:

We added extra cheese and meat (both 0/0), so this is a satisfying morning meal. Plus, you can wrap it up and take it on the road.

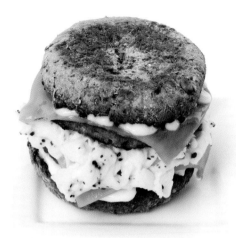

Savory Breakfast Sandwich

Serves 4

8 breakfast sausage patties
8 whole eggs
¼ cup half-and-half
1 Tbsp. butter
4 Rudi's Organic Bakery Whole Grain
    Wheat English Muffins
8 slices cheddar cheese
4 Tbsp. mayonnaise

1. Cook the sausage according to package directions; set aside.

2. Whisk the eggs with half-and-half, and season to taste. Melt the butter in a large skillet over medium heat. Add the egg mixture to a pan, and scramble until just cooked through.

3. Toast the English muffins, then spread each side with mayonnaise. Build each sandwich with the bottom muffin, and top with 1 slice of cheese, 1 sausage patty, ¼ of the egg mixture, 1 sausage patty, and 1 slice of cheese. Place the other half of the muffin on top.

4. Serve 1 sandwich per person.

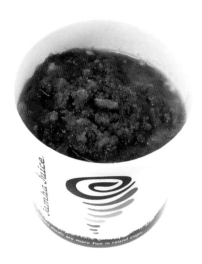

BELLY BAD

S/C Value = 25/3

BELLY GOOD

S/C Value = 1/2

Jamba Juice Apple Cinnamon Oatmeal

This oatmeal is topped with compote, which is fruit and sugar combined over heat until it becomes slightly syrupy. Watch out for any kind of compote, as it's guaranteed to be loaded with sugar.

Apple Cinnamon Oatmeal Do-Over:

Add stevia to plain oatmeal; the flavored ones overdo it on sugar. You can add cinnamon as well—it's a powerful antioxidant.

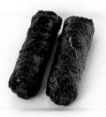
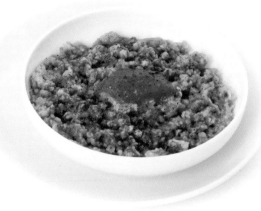

Sweet Apricot Oatmeal

Oatmeal:
½ cup Quaker Instant Oatmeal Original
1 packet of stevia
1 Tbsp. Nature's Hollow Sugar Free Apricot
    Preserves
¼ tsp. cinnamon
1 Tbsp. chopped pecans

Other sides:
2 sausage links

1. For the oatmeal: Prepare oats with water according to package instructions. Put the cooked oatmeal in a bowl; sweeten with stevia to taste and swirl in the apricot preserves. Sprinkle with cinnamon and pecans.

2. For the sausage links: Cook as directed.

3. Serve the oatmeal with the sausage links.

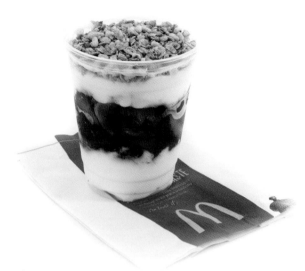

BELLY BAD

S/C Value = 21/2

BELLY GOOD

S/C Value = 5/2

McDonald's Fruit 'n Yogurt Parfait

With 21 grams of sugar, this isn't the healthy snack you think it is. You're better off grabbing a Sausage McMuffin—with 2 grams of sugar and 29 carbs, it has an S/C value of just 2/2.

Fruit 'n Yogurt Parfait Do-Over:

Yogurt is a great source of probiotics, which are critical for your digestive health and can help your body get rid of waste.

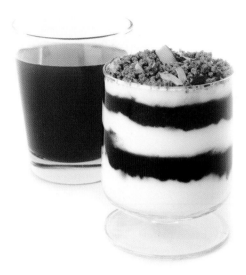

Lovely Layered Parfait

Serves 1

Parfait:

2 Tbsp. frozen raspberries, unsweetened

1 Tbsp. Nature's Hollow Sugar Free Raspberry Preserves

2 Tbsp. frozen blackberries, unsweetened

1 Tbsp. Nature's Hollow Sugar Free Wild Blueberry Preserves

⅓ cup FAGE Total Yogurt (Classic, 0%, 2%, or 5%)

2 Tbsp. Food for Life Ezekiel 4:9 Almond Cereal

Other sides:

Nature's Plus Source of Life Red Lightning drink

1. For the parfait: Mix the raspberries with raspberry preserves in a bowl, and mix the blackberries with blueberry preserves in a separate bowl. Build the parfait by layering yogurt, blackberry mix, yogurt, raspberry mix, yogurt. Top with cereal.

2. For the drink: Mix with water according to package instructions.

3. Serve the parfait with the drink.

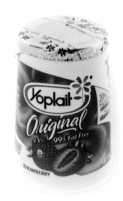

BELLY BAD	BELLY GOOD
S/C Value = 27/2	S/C Value = 4/1

Yoplait Original Strawberry Yogurt

This little yogurt holds almost 2 days' worth of sugar on the Belly Fat Cure. Avoid "light" versions, too—most contain aspartame, an artificial sweetener that is an excitotoxin.

Strawberry Yogurt Do-Over:

Always use Greek yogurt like the FAGE brand because it's lower in sugar than regular yogurt.

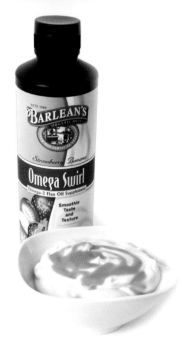

Strawberry Swirl Yogurt

Serves 1

½ cup FAGE Total Yogurt (Classic, 0%, 2%, or 5%)

2 Tbsp. Barlean's Strawberry Banana Omega Swirl

1. Put the yogurt into a small bowl.

2. Swirl Barlean's onto the yogurt and serve.

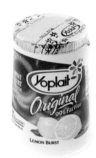

BELLY BAD

S/C Value = 31/2

Yoplait Original Lemon Burst Yogurt

Be wary of foods labeled "fat free"—they have to make up for taste somehow, and they do so mostly by adding sugar or artificial sweeteners.

BELLY GOOD

S/C Value = 4/1

Lemon Yogurt Do-Over:

Barlean's Lemon Zest Omega Swirl is actually made of fish oil, a healthy source of omega-3s— this is truly a remarkable, indulgent dream.

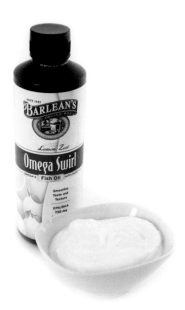

Tart Lemon Yogurt

Serves 1

½ cup FAGE Total Yogurt (Classic, 0%, 2%, or 5%)
1 Tbsp. Barlean's Lemon Zest Omega Swirl

1. Put the yogurt into a small bowl.

2. Swirl Barlean's onto the yogurt and serve.

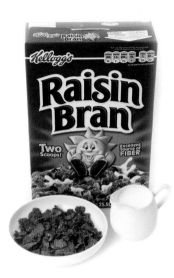

BELLY BAD

S/C Value = 31/3

BELLY GOOD

S/C Value = 3/2

Kellogg's Raisin Bran with Milk

This cereal alone has 19 grams of sugar in a serving—almost 5 tsp! Raisins are particularly high in sugar since the drying process raises the amount of grapes' natural sugars.

Cereal with Milk Do-Over:

One serving of U.S. Mills Uncle Sam Cereal has less than 1 gram of sugar, yet it has 10 grams of fiber—a great start to your day.

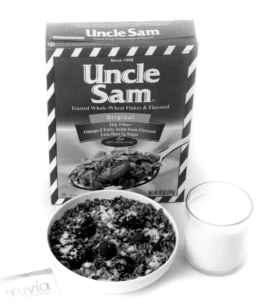

Berry Sweet Cereal

Serves 1

½ cup U.S. Mills Uncle Sam Cereal Original
1 packet approved sweetener
2 raspberries
4 blackberries
½ cup Almond Breeze Original Unsweetened
    Almond Milk

1. Pour the cereal into a bowl and sprinkle with sweetener and berries. Add almond milk and serve.

CARB SWAP

CEREALS

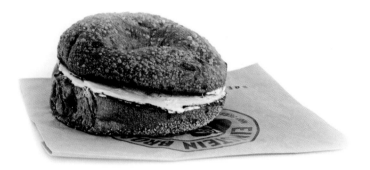

BELLY BAD

S/C Value = 14/4

Einstein Bros. Cinnamon Raisin Bagel with Whipped Plain Cream Cheese

The S/C Value gives you 6 servings of carbs per day— this single bagel takes away 4 of those servings. On top of that, it has almost a whole day's worth of sugar.

BELLY GOOD

S/C Value = 3/2

Bagel Breakfast Do-Over:

Smoked salmon has more than 20 grams of protein in 1 serving. Plus, salmon is a fatty, cold-water fish, so it's rich in omega-3 fatty acids.

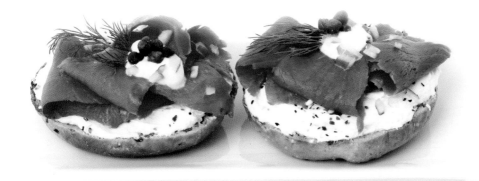

Luscious Lox Bagel

Serves 4

4 Rudi's Organic Bakery Multigrain Bagels
8 Tbsp. Kraft Philadelphia Cream Cheese, softened
4 Tbsp. diced red onion
2 Tbsp. capers, drained
1 Tbsp. Lawry's Lemon Pepper, or Mrs. Dash Original Blend
2 tsp. fresh lemon juice
16 oz. smoked salmon
4 tsp. sour cream
8 sprigs fresh dill

1. Toast the bagels and lay them out open-faced.

2. Mix the cream cheese with diced onions, capers, seasonings, and lemon juice. Reserve a few capers for garnish.

3. Spread each bagel side with 1 Tbsp. cream-cheese mixture; top with 2 oz. salmon.

4. Garnish each with ½ tsp. of sour cream, as well as some fresh dill and reserved capers.

5. Serve 2 halves per person.

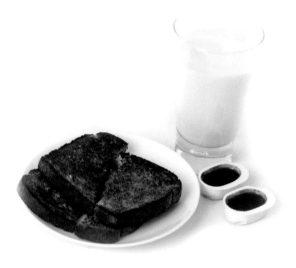

BELLY BAD

S/C Value = 28/3

Denny's Toast with Jam and Milk

Most sugars get processed in your liver and converted to fat in your blood, creating high cholesterol. The next time you're at Denny's, try having toast with peanut butter and a cup of coffee.

BELLY GOOD

S/C Value = 3/2

Toast with Jam and Milk Do-Over:

Oroweat Light 100% Whole Wheat Bread is available nationwide and isn't made with high-fructose corn syrup (unlike other major brands).

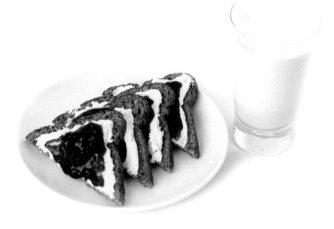

Indulgent Cream-Cheese Toast

Serves 1

Toast:
2 slices Oroweat Light 100% Whole Wheat Bread
2 Tbsp. Kraft Philadelphia Cream Cheese
2 Tbsp. Nature's Hollow Sugar Free Preserves
  (any flavor)

Other sides:
8 oz. Almond Breeze Original Unsweetened
  Almond Milk

1. Toast the bread. Spread with the cream cheese, then top with preserves.

2. Slice diagonally and serve with a glass of almond milk.

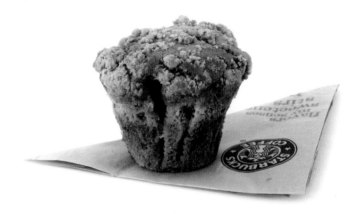

BELLY BAD

S/C Value = 33/3

BELLY GOOD

S/C Value = 0/2

Starbucks Blueberry Streusel Muffin

This muffin from Starbucks has more sugar than 3 Krispy Kreme doughnuts. Next time you're at Starbucks, opt for a bagel or mixed nuts as a snack with your coffee.

Blueberry Muffin Do-Over:

By using the sugar alcohol xylitol, you can have 2 muffins with butter and Nature's Hollow Sugar Free Preserves, and you will not have eaten *any* sugar. Amazing!

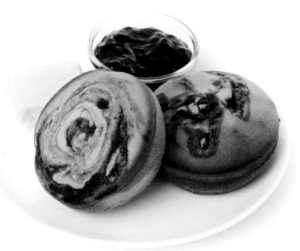

Blueberry Velvet Muffins

Serves 6

Muffin:
Cooking spray
2 cups Arrowhead Mills Organic Soy Flour
2 tsp. baking powder
¼ tsp. salt
⅓ cup powdered xylitol
4 eggs
⅔ cup water
½ cup butter, melted
4 Tbsp. Nature's Hollow Sugar Free Wild
    Blueberry Preserves

Other sides:
6 Tbsp. Nature's Hollow Sugar Free Wild
    Blueberry Preserves, for serving
6 pats butter

1. For the muffins: Preheat oven to 350° F. Coat a 12-muffin tin with cooking spray. Sift dry ingredients together in a large mixing bowl. In a small bowl, whisk together the eggs and water; stir in melted butter. Make a well in the center of the dry ingredients and pour in the wet ingredients. Mix until combined. Fill the muffin cups ⅔ full, and top each with 1 tsp. preserves; swirl preserves slightly with a toothpick. Bake for about 15 minutes or until a toothpick or tester comes away clean.

2. Serve 2 muffins per person with a pat of butter and a side of preserves.

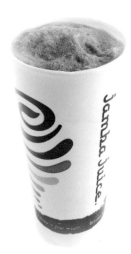

BELLY BAD

S/C Value = 84/5

BELLY GOOD

S/C Value = 0/1

Jamba Juice Chocolate Moo'd Smoothie

I think that the shocking number on this smoothie speaks for itself—84 grams of sugar! And that's for the 16-oz. size; the original 24-oz. version has a whopping 120 grams.

Chocolate Smoothie Do-Over:

If you don't have time to make whipped cream (just a few minutes), try any non-fat whipped topping made with a sugar alcohol.

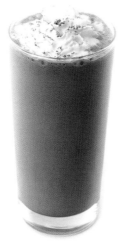

Chocolate Lovers' Shake

Serves 1

Shake:
1 scoop (30 grams) Jay Robb Chocolate Whey
  Protein Powder
½ cup Clemmy's Vanilla Bean Ice Cream
  (see page 297)
½ cup Almond Breeze Vanilla Unsweetened
  Almond Milk
½ packet Truvia

Whipped topping:
¼ cup cold whipping cream
1 packet Truvia

1. For the shake: Combine all listed ingredients in a blender and process until smooth.

2. For the whipped topping: Whip the cream with sweetener until soft peaks form.

3. Pour the shake into a glass and top with whipped cream. Garnish with a pinch of chocolate protein powder.

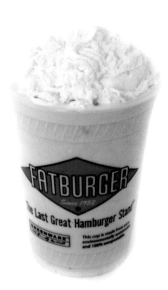

BELLY BAD

S/C Value = 85/6

BELLY GOOD

S/C Value = 3/2

Fatburger Strawberry Shake

With 85 grams of sugar, this shake has nearly 6 days' worth of sugar on the Belly Fat Cure—and it covers all of your carbs for the entire day.

Strawberry Shake Do-Over:

Strawberries are an excellent source of vitamin C: 8 medium berries provide 160% of the RDA for this essential vitamin—all for under 5 grams of sugar.

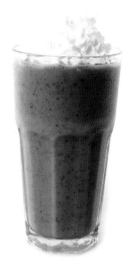

Sweet Strawberry Smoothie

Serves 1

Smoothie:
½ cup frozen unsweetened strawberries
½ cup Clemmy's Vanilla Bean Ice Cream
(see page 297)
½ cup Almond Breeze Vanilla Unsweetened
Almond Milk
½ packet Truvia

Whipped topping:
¼ cup cold whipping cream
1 packet Truvia

1. For the smoothie: Combine all listed ingredients in a blender and process until smooth.

2. For the whipped topping: Whip the cream with sweetener until soft peaks form.

3. Pour the smoothie into a glass and top with whipped cream.

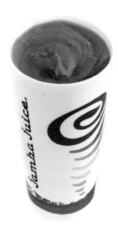

BELLY BAD

S/C Value = 85/6

BELLY GOOD

S/C Value = 1/2

Jamba Juice Peanut Butter Moo'd Smoothie

With 75 grams, this smoothie from Jamba Juice has *5* days' worth of sugar on the Belly Fat Cure—that's more than a strawberry milkshake from Baskin-Robbins.

Peanut Butter Smoothie Do-Over:

Look for peanut butter with simple ingredients. Laura Scudder's contains only peanuts and salt. It also has just 1 gram of sugar per serving.

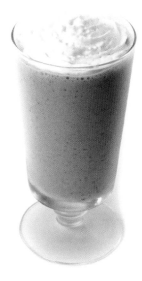

Go Nutty Shake

Serves 1

Shake:
1 scoop (30 grams) Jay Robb Whey Protein
Powder
½ cup Clemmy's Vanilla Bean Ice Cream
(see page 297)
½ cup Almond Breeze Vanilla Unsweetened
Almond Milk
2 Tbsp. Laura Scudder's All Natural Old
Fashioned Smooth Peanut Butter
½ packet Truvia

Whipped topping:
¼ cup cold whipping cream
1 packet Truvia

1. For the shake: Combine all listed ingredients in a blender and process until smooth.

2. For the whipped topping: Whip the cream with sweetener until soft peaks form.

3. Pour the shake into a glass and top with whipped cream.

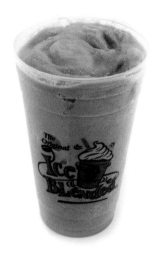

BELLY BAD

S/C Value = 71/5

The Coffee Bean & Tea Leaf Pomegranate Blueberry Ice Blended

The 71 grams of sugar in this drink will drag your immune system down by paralyzing your white blood cells, and it will make sure you *gain* belly fat, not lose it.

BELLY GOOD

S/C Value = 2/2

Pomegranate Blueberry Ice Blended Do-Over:

Raspberries and blackberries are rich in phytonutrients, which help the body fight off oxidation, a process that causes aging through the release of free radicals.

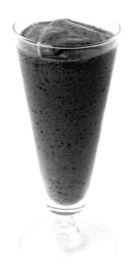

Frosty Berry Shake

Serves 1

½ cup Clemmy's Vanilla Bean Ice Cream (see page 297)
½ cup Almond Breeze Vanilla Unsweetened Almond Milk
1 Tbsp. Nature's Hollow Sugar Free Mountain Berry Preserves
2 Tbsp. frozen raspberries
2 Tbsp. frozen blackberries
1½ Tbsp. Barlean's Pomegranate Blueberry Total Omega Vegan Swirl

1. Combine all of the ingredients in a blender and process until smooth.

2. Pour the shake into a glass and serve.

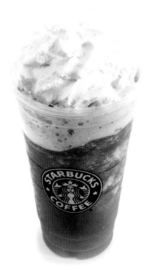

BELLY BAD

S/C Value = 47/3

BELLY GOOD

S/C Value = 0/1

Starbucks Mocha Frappuccino

If you want a cool drink
from Starbucks,
opt for an iced coffee
and add a little
half-and-half—delicious!

Mocha Frappuccino Do-Over:

Make this recipe extra easy
by freezing coffee in
ice-cube trays ahead of
time; this cuts out your
coffee brewing time.

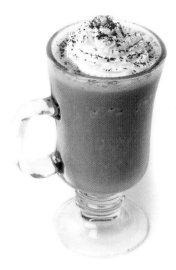

Perky Blended Coffee Shake

Serves 1

Shake:
1 cup ice
½ cup cold coffee
2 tsp. heavy cream
1 scoop (30 grams) Jay Robb Vanilla Whey
    Protein Powder
1 packet Truvia

Whipped topping:
¼ cup cold whipping cream
1 packet Truvia
1 pinch cocoa powder

1. For the shake: Combine all listed ingredients in a blender and process until smooth.

2. For the whipped topping: Whip the cream with sweetener until soft peaks form.

3. Pour the shake into a glass and top with whipped cream. Dust with cocoa powder.

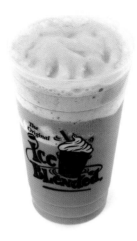

BELLY BAD

S/C Value = 59/4

BELLY GOOD

S/C Value = 0/1

The Coffee Bean & Tea Leaf Vanilla Ice Blended

Nearly every blended drink on Coffee Bean's menu has double-digit sugar grams (some even have *triple* digits); opt for an unsweetened iced tea or iced coffee instead.

Vanilla Ice Blended Do-Over:

Lipton flavored teas add great flavor without any sugar. They can also be brewed extra strong and put on ice for a refreshing cold drink.

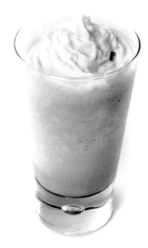

Silky Vanilla Drink

Serves 1

Drink:
2 tea bags, vanilla flavored
½ cup boiling water
1 packet Truvia
1 cup ice
¼ cup heavy cream
1 scoop (30 grams) Jay Robb Vanilla Whey
    Protein Powder

Whipped topping:
¼ cup cold whipping cream
1 packet Truvia

1. For the drink: Pour boiling water over the tea bags; allow to steep for 5 minutes. Remove tea bags and carefully squeeze, then stir in sweetener; chill. Blend the chilled tea mixture with the next three ingredients.

2. For the whipped topping: Whip cream with sweetener until soft peaks form.

3. Pour the drink into a glass and top with whipped cream.

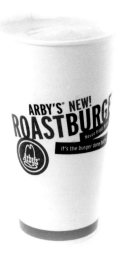

BELLY BAD

S/C Value = 95/5

Arby's Jamocha Swirl Shake

"Mocha" originally described coffee coming from the city of Mocha in Yemen. Now it describes any chocolate-flavored coffee and is considered one of the most popular varieties—skip this Jamocha version.

BELLY GOOD

S/C Value = 0/1

Jamocha Swirl Shake Do-Over:

Here I used Jay Robb Chocolate Whey Protein Powder, sweetened with Truvia, and added another packet to the whipped topping for an extra treat.

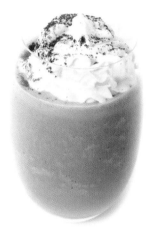

Magical Mocha Blend

Serves 1

Shake:

1 cup ice

½ cup cold coffee

2 tsp. heavy cream

1 scoop (30 grams) Jay Robb Chocolate
    Whey Protein Powder

1 packet Truvia

Whipped topping:

¼ cup cold whipping cream

1 packet Truvia

1 pinch cocoa powder

1. For the shake: Combine all listed ingredients in a blender and process until smooth.

2. For the whipped topping: Whip the cream with sweetener until soft peaks form.

3. Pour the shake into a glass and top with whipped cream. Dust with cocoa powder.

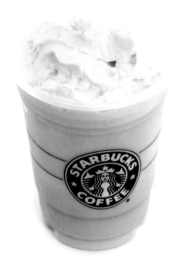

BELLY BAD

S/C Value = 69/5

Starbucks Tazo Green Tea Frappuccino Blended Crème

The description says that it's only "lightly sweetened," but there's nothing light about this amount of sugar; in fact, it's almost 5 days' worth of sugar on the Belly Fat Cure.

BELLY GOOD

S/C Value = 1/1

Green Tea Frappuccino Blended Crème Do-Over:

Green and black teas come from the same tea leaves, but black tea is fermented longer and loses phytochemicals, the antioxidant properties found in tea.

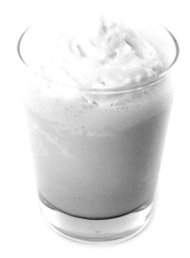

Energize Me Green Tea

Serves 1

Tea:
2 green-tea bags
½ cup boiling water
1 packet Truvia
1 cup ice
¼ cup heavy cream
1 scoop (30 grams) Jay Robb Vanilla
    Whey Protein Powder

Whipped topping:
¼ cup cold whipping cream
1 packet Truvia

1. For the tea: Pour boiling water over the tea bags; allow to steep for 5 minutes. Remove tea bags and carefully squeeze, then stir in sweetener; chill. Combine the chilled tea mixture with the next three ingredients in a blender, and process until smooth.

2. For the whipped topping: Whip cream with sweetener until soft peaks form.

3. Pour the drink into a glass and top with whipped cream.

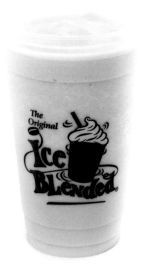

BELLY BAD

S/C Value = 94/6

BELLY GOOD

S/C Value = 0/1

The Coffee Bean & Tea Leaf Banana Caramel Ice Blended

The average daily sugar consumption is 189 grams a day. This drink is almost half of that by itself—add 2 sodas and you've just about reached that number in beverages alone.

Banana Caramel Ice Blended Do-Over:

Sugar alcohols such as xylitol (found in the Seelect Teas' Organic Caramel Syrup used in this drink) don't cause tooth decay; in fact, xylitol has even been shown to help prevent cavities.

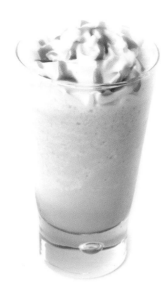

Smooth Caramel Truffle Drink

Serves 1

Drink:
2 Lipton Vanilla Caramel Truffle Tea Bags
½ cup boiling water
1 packet Truvia
1 scoop (30 grams) Jay Robb Vanilla Whey
    Protein Powder
2 Tbsp. heavy cream
¼ cup ice

Whipped topping:
¼ cup cold whipping cream
1 packet Truvia
1 Tbsp. Seelect Teas' Organic Caramel Syrup

1. For the drink: Pour boiling water over the tea bags; cover and brew 5 minutes. Remove tea bags and squeeze, then stir in sweetener; chill. Blend all ingredients in a blender until smooth.

2. For the whipped topping: Whip cream with sweetener until soft peaks form.

3. Pour the drink into a glass and top with whipped cream and caramel syrup.

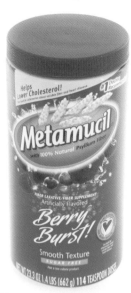

BELLY BAD

S/C Value = 0/1

BELLY GOOD

S/C Value = 0/2

Metamucil Berry Burst! Fiber Drink

The S/C Value is 0/1, but there are two concerns here: aspartame and acesulfame potassium. Recent studies have shown that aspartame use can cause an accumulation of formaldehyde in the brain. Acesulfame potassium contains the carcinogen methylene chloride.

Fiber Drink Do-Over:

Taking probiotics with this shake, which has approximately 10 grams of fiber, will ensure a healthy digestive system and accelerate false belly fat loss.

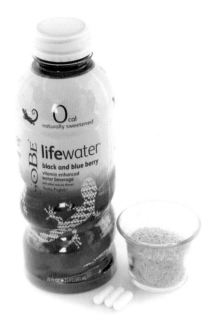

Belly Fat Cure Drink

Serves 1

Drink:

1 (20-oz.) bottle of SoBe Lifewater
    (any PureVia-sweetened flavor)
2½ Tbsp. psyllium husks
3 probiotic capsules

1. Mix the psyllium husks with water.

2. Take the probiotics with the shake, and drink remainder immediately.

Note: I'm using SoBe Black and Blue Berry Lifewater, but feel free to use 20 oz. of plain water or any beverage listed on page 289.

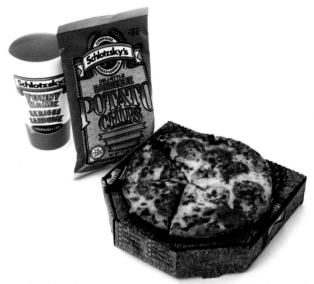

BELLY BAD

S/C Value = 52/8

Schlotzsky's Pepperoni & Double Cheese Pizza Meal Deal

This meal has 8 servings of carbs—more than you should have in an entire day. Also, strawberry lemonade actually has more sugar than soda; try sparkling water with a squeeze of lemon instead.

BELLY GOOD

S/C Value = 4/2

Pepperoni Pizza Meal
Do-Over:

Enjoy this with some fresh arugula.
One of my favorite greens, it is rich in vitamins and minerals and an excellent source of antioxidants.

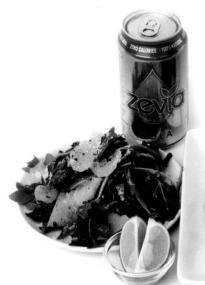
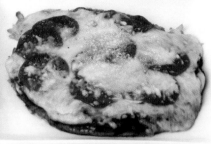

Savory Pepperoni Pizza

Serves 4

Pizza:
4 (6") Sara Lee Mr. Pita Whole Wheat Pita Breads
8 Tbsp. Ragú Homemade Style Pizza Sauce
1 cup grated mozzarella
12 oz. sliced pepperoni
1 Tbsp. grated Parmesan

Salad:
4 cups arugula greens
1 lime, cut into wedges
16 (1") pieces of shaved Parmesan

Other sides:
4 cans Zevia Natural Cola

1. For the pizza: Preheat oven to 425° F. Warm pitas on a baking sheet in the oven for 5 minutes; remove.

2. Spread 2 Tbsp. of pizza sauce over each pita; top with cheese and pepperoni. Bake for 8–10 minutes or until cheese has melted. Garnish with grated Parmesan.

3. For the salad: Shave Parmesan cheese with a vegetable peeler over the arugula and garnish with fresh lime wedges.

4. Serve with 1 soda per person.

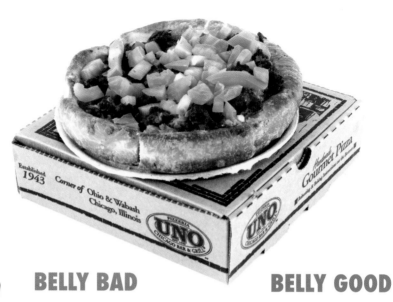

BELLY BAD

S/C Value = 6/6

BELLY GOOD

S/C Value = 3/2

Uno Chicago Grill Bacon, Cheddar & Tomato Deep Dish Pizza (indiv. size)

Formerly known as Pizzeria Uno, then Uno, this chain popularized deep-dish pizza in this country. That deep dish helps this pizza take up all of your carbs for the day.

Bacon, Cheddar & Tomato Pizza Do-Over:

I used Amy's Organic Family Marinara Pasta Sauce for this pizza, which adds a nice flavor (I love Amy's because the company uses all-natural ingredients).

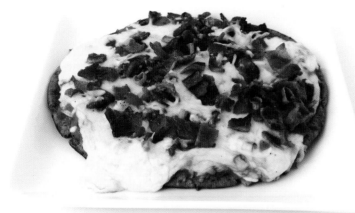

Crispy Bacon Pizza

Serves 4

4 (6") Sara Lee Mr. Pita Whole Wheat Pita Breads
8 Tbsp. Amy's Organic Family Marinara Pasta
  Sauce
1 cup shredded Italian blend or pizza blend
  cheese
8 strips of bacon, cooked and roughly chopped
2 green onions, green parts only, thinly sliced
½ cup diced tomatoes
Grated Parmesan, for serving
Red chili flakes, for serving

1. Preheat oven to 425° F. Warm pitas on a baking sheet in the oven for 5 minutes; remove.

2. Spread 2 Tbsp. of the pasta sauce over each pita; top with cheese, bacon, green onions, and tomatoes.

3. Bake for 8–10 minutes or until cheese is melted. Garnish with Parmesan and red chili flakes to taste.

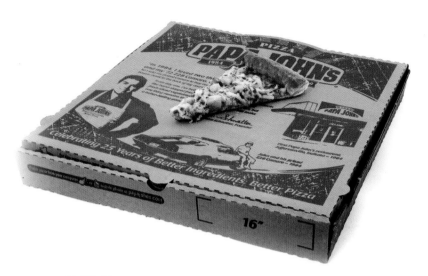

BELLY BAD

S/C Value = 8/3

BELLY GOOD

S/C Value = 2/2

Papa John's Hawaiian BBQ Chicken Pizza

Two of the high-sugar culprits here are barbecue sauce and pineapple. Some popular brands of barbecue sauce have as much as 12 grams of sugar in just 2 Tbsp.

BBQ Chicken Pizza Do-Over:

We used Scott's Barbecue Sauce, which is both sugar and fat free and contains just a few simple ingredients: vinegar, peppers, salt, spices, and water.

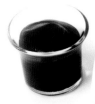
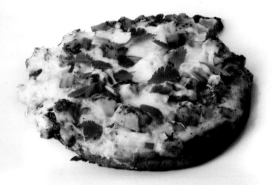

Robust BBQ Chicken Pizza

Serves 4

Pizza:
4 (6") Sara Lee Mr. Pita Whole Wheat Pita Breads
8 Tbsp. Scott's Barbecue Sauce
¾ cup grated smoked Gouda cheese
½ cup grated mozzarella
2 chicken breasts, cooked and shredded
2½ Tbsp. diced red onion
2 Tbsp. chopped fresh cilantro, for garnish

Other sides:
½ cup Scott's Barbecue Sauce, for serving

1. Preheat oven to 425° F. Warm pitas on a baking sheet in the oven for 5 minutes; remove.

2. Spread 2 Tbsp. of barbecue sauce over each pita; top with cheese, chicken, and red onions.

3. Bake for 8–10 minutes or until cheese is melted. Remove and garnish with cilantro to taste.

4. Serve with a side of barbecue sauce.

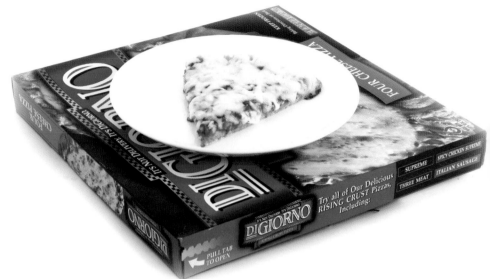

BELLY BAD

S/C Value = 8/2

DiGiorno Four Cheese Pizza

Under all that cheese is a high-sugar tomato sauce; just 1 slice of pizza has 8 grams of sugar. It may be quick to make, but it will also quickly add belly fat.

BELLY GOOD

S/C Value = 2/2

Four Cheese Pizza Do-Over:

Use Mr. Pita Whole Wheat Pita Bread by Sara Lee and enjoy your pizza without any guilt.

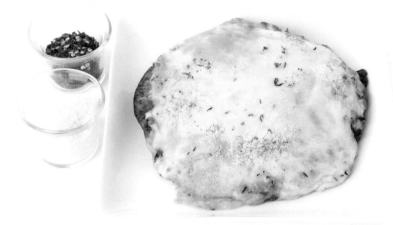

Quattro Formaggio Pizza

Serves 4

4 (6") Sara Lee Mr. Pita Whole Wheat Pita Breads
8 Tbsp. Seeds of Change Romagna Three
   Cheese Pasta Sauce
½ cup grated mozzarella
½ cup grated provolone
½ cup grated fontina
½ cup grated Parmesan
2 Tbsp. chopped fresh basil
Grated Parmesan, for serving
Red chili flakes, for serving

1. Preheat oven to 425° F. Warm pitas on a baking sheet in the oven for 5 minutes; remove.

2. Spread 2 Tbsp. of pasta sauce over each pita; top each with cheese.

3. Bake for 8–10 minutes or until cheese is melted. Garnish with fresh basil.

4. Serve with a side of chili flakes and Parmesan to taste.

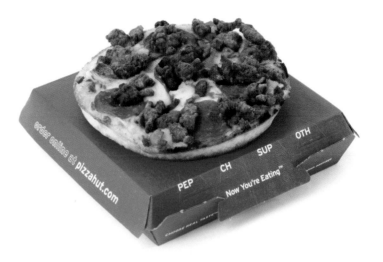

BELLY BAD

S/C Value = 7/4

BELLY GOOD

S/C Value = 2/2

Pizza Hut Meat Lover's Personal Pan Pizza

Most of Pizza Hut's
personal pizzas have
at least 7 grams of sugar;
choose their All American
Traditional wings instead.

(Nutritional information is
available at **pizzahut.com**.)

Meat Lover's Pizza Do-Over:

I'm using a pasta sauce
from Seeds of Change
called Marinara
di Venezia—with 0 grams
of sugar, you can't
go wrong with it.

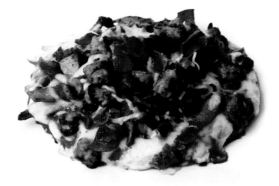

Mouthwatering Meaty Pizza

Serves 4

4 oz. Italian sausage, sweet or hot, casings
   removed
4 (6") Sara Lee Mr. Pita Whole Wheat Pita Bread
8 Tbsp. Seeds of Change Marinara di Venezia
   Pasta Sauce
1 cup grated mozzarella
4 oz. sliced pepperoni
4 slices Canadian bacon, diced
Grated Parmesan, to taste
Red chili flakes, to taste

1. Preheat oven to 425° F. In a medium skillet over medium heat, brown sausage, breaking it up with the back of a wooden spoon. When cooked, discard fat and set sausage aside. Warm pitas on a baking sheet in the oven for 5 minutes; remove.

2. Spread 2 Tbsp. of pasta sauce over each pita; top with cheese, sausage, pepperoni, and Canadian bacon.

3. Bake for 8–10 minutes or until cheese is melted.

4. Serve grated Parmesan and red chili flakes on the side.

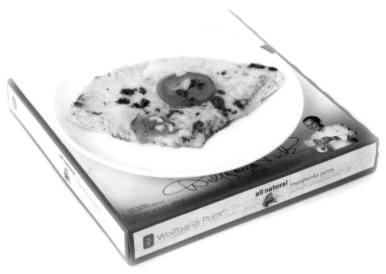

BELLY BAD

S/C Value = 9/2

BELLY GOOD

S/C Value = 3/2

Wolfgang Puck All-Natural Margherita Pizza

While Wolfgang Puck does use all-natural ingredients, this frozen pizza has too much sugar if you want to lose belly fat and be healthy.

Margherita Pizza Do-Over:

Tomatoes are an excellent source of the phytonutrient lycopene, which gives them their bright red color and has proven cancer-fighting benefits.

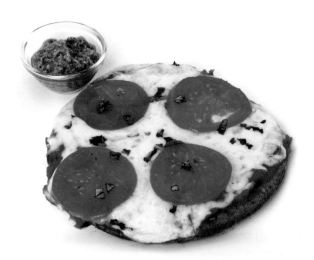

Tasty Margherita Pizza

Serves 4

Pizza:
4 (6") Sara Lee Mr. Pita Whole Wheat Pita Breads
8 Tbsp. Seeds of Change Tomato Basil
   Genovese Pasta Sauce
Salt and pepper, to taste
1 tsp. dried oregano
12 oz. fresh mozzarella, sliced
16 Roma tomato slices
8 basil leaves, torn
Extra-virgin olive oil, to drizzle
4 Tbsp. grated Parmesan

Other sides:
8 Tbsp. DeLallo Pesto

1. Preheat oven to 425° F. Warm pitas on a baking sheet in the oven for 5 minutes; remove.

2. Spread 2 Tbsp. of pasta sauce over each pita; sprinkle with salt, pepper, and oregano. Arrange sliced mozzarella, tomato slices, and basil leaves over the top. Drizzle with olive oil and sprinkle with Parmesan.

3. Bake for 8–10 minutes or until cheese is melted.

4. Serve with a side of pesto.

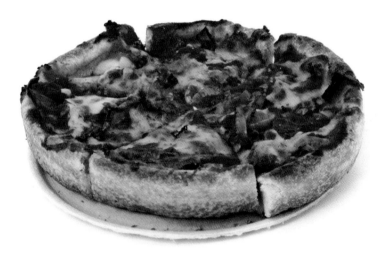

BELLY BAD

S/C Value = 12/9

BELLY GOOD

S/C Value = 2/2

Uno Chicago Grill Veggie Deep Dish Pizza

Veggie pizza can taste great and be healthy at the same time, but this version from Uno Chicago Grill goes overboard on sugar and carbs. Aim for a 5/2 or less at each meal.

Veggie Pizza Do-Over:

Broccoli is one of the smartest veggie choices: it's a good source of calcium, vitamin C, beta-carotene, and fiber, to name just a few of its benefits.

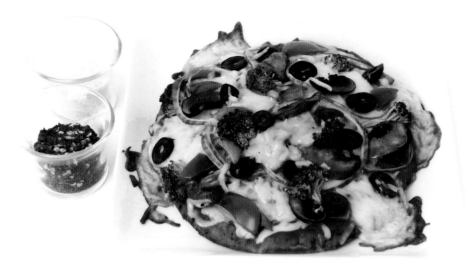

Very Veggie Pizza

Serves 4

4 (6") Sara Lee Mr. Pita Whole Wheat Pita Breads
½ cup Seeds of Change Tomato Basil
    Genovese Pasta Sauce
1 cup grated mozzarella
½ red onion, thinly sliced
1 cup sliced mushrooms
1 cup chopped broccoli florets
¼ cup diced green pepper
1 (6-oz.) can sliced black olives, drained
Salt and pepper, to taste
1 tsp. Italian seasoning
Grated Parmesan, for serving
Red chili flakes, for serving

1. Preheat oven to 425° F. Warm pitas on a baking sheet in the oven for 5 minutes; remove.

2. Spread 2 Tbsp. of pasta sauce over each pita; top with cheese and vegetables. Sprinkle with salt, pepper, and oregano.

3. Bake for 8–10 minutes or until cheese is melted.

4. Serve with grated Parmesan and red chili flakes on the side.

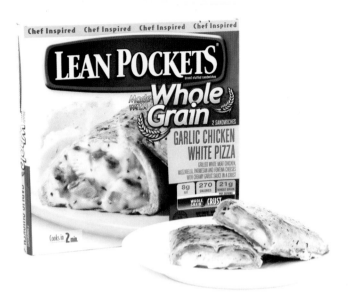

BELLY BAD

S/C Value = 9/2

BELLY GOOD

S/C Value = 2/2

Lean Pockets Garlic Chicken White Pizza

Lean Pockets gets credit for using whole-wheat flour, but it has almost a full day's supply of sugar. Pass on this one.

Garlic Chicken Pizza Do-Over:

It's called a "white pizza" because it has no tomato sauce like other types of pizza. Instead, Alfredo sauce is used.

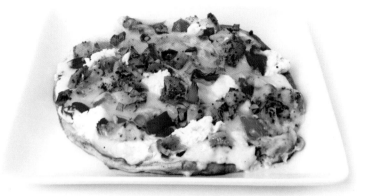

Pizza Blanca

Serves 4

4 (6") Sara Lee Mr. Pita Whole Wheat Pita Breads
8 Tbsp. Classico Creamy Alfredo Sauce
1 cup shredded mozzarella
2 chicken breasts, cooked and shredded
½ cup jarred roasted yellow and red
    peppers, diced
Salt and pepper, to taste
½ cup ricotta cheese
¼ cup basil, torn
Grated Parmesan, for serving
Red chili flakes, for serving

1. Preheat oven to 425° F. Warm pitas on a baking sheet in the oven for 5 minutes; remove.

2. Spread 2 Tbsp. of Alfredo sauce over each pita; top with chicken, peppers, and mozzarella. Drop ricotta by the teaspoon evenly over pitas. Season with salt and pepper, and sprinkle with torn basil.

3. Bake for 8–10 minutes or until cheese is melted.

4. Serve with grated Parmesan and red chili flakes on the side.

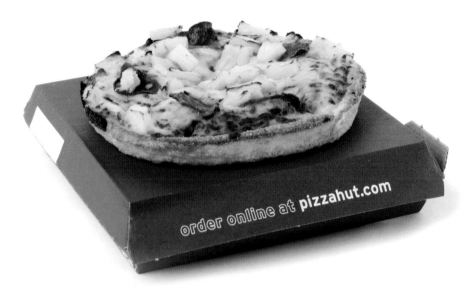

order online at **pizzahut.com**

BELLY BAD

S/C Value = 9/4

Pizza Hut Quartered Ham and Pineapple Personal Pan Pizza

Pizza Hut is the "world's largest user of cheese." I love cheese, but not when it comes with 9 grams of sugar, like this ham and pineapple pizza does.

BELLY GOOD

S/C Value = 5/2

Ham and Pineapple Pizza Do-Over:

Contrary to its name, Hawaiian pizza doesn't actually come from Hawaii. It's believed to have been adapted from a German sandwich called "Toast Hawaii."

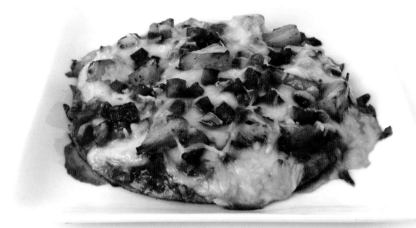

Sweet Hawaiian Pizza

Serves 4

4 (6") Sara Lee Mr. Pita Whole Wheat Pita Breads
8 Tbsp. Seeds of Change Marinara di Venezia
   Pasta Sauce
⅓ cup shredded mozzarella
1 cup shredded Monterey Jack or pepper Jack
   cheese
2 cups diced baked ham or chopped deli ham
1 cup diced pineapple

1. Preheat oven to 425° F. Warm pitas on a baking sheet in the oven for 5 minutes; remove.

2. Spread 2 Tbsp. of pasta sauce over each pita; top with cheese, ham, and pineapple.

3. Bake for 8–10 minutes or until cheese is melted, and serve.

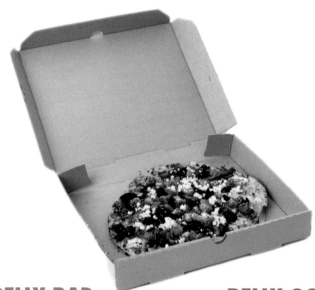

BELLY BAD

S/C Value = 6/5

BELLY GOOD

S/C Value = 5/2

Uno Chicago Grill Mediterranean Flatbread Pizza

Typically, flatbreads don't "rise" like other types of bread, so they're often a bit lighter. The kind used in this dish, however, has 5 carb servings, which is far from light.

Mediterranean Flatbread Pizza Do-Over:

With all of its classic Mediterranean flavors, this is perfect for a quick spring or summer meal— enjoy it on the patio with sparkling water with lime.

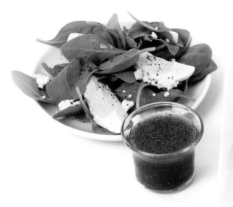
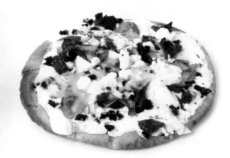

Superb Greek Pizza

Serves 4

Pizza:
4 (6") Sara Lee Mr. Pita Whole Wheat Pita Breads
8 Tbsp. Classico Creamy Alfredo Sauce
1 cup crumbled feta cheese
½ cup pitted Kalamata olives
2½ Tbsp. diced red onion
¼ cup sun-dried tomatoes, roughly chopped
¼ cup basil leaves, torn

Salad:
12 oz. baby spinach leaves
2 hard-boiled eggs, chopped
½ cup crumbled feta cheese
⅓ cup extra-virgin olive oil
2 Tbsp. red-wine vinegar
Salt and pepper, to taste

1. For the pizza: Preheat oven to 425° F. Warm pitas on a baking sheet in the oven for 5 minutes; remove.

2. Spread 2 Tbsp. of Alfredo sauce over each pita; top with feta, olives, onions, and tomatoes; sprinkle with torn basil. Bake for 8–10 minutes or until heated through.

3. For the salad: Divide the spinach, eggs, and feta onto four chilled salad plates.

4. In a small bowl, whisk together the olive oil and red-wine vinegar; dress salads. Season with salt and pepper to taste.

5. Serve the pizza and salad.

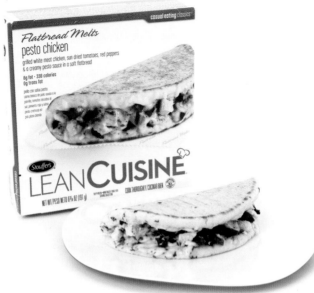

BELLY BAD

S/C Value = 6/3

BELLY GOOD

S/C Value = 3/2

Lean Cuisine Pesto Chicken Flatbread Melts

Lean Cuisine Flatbread Melts might look good, but this pesto version is too high in sugar and carbs for a single meal on the Belly Fat Cure.

Pesto Chicken Flatbread Melt Do-Over:

Basil can be used as a garnish on just about any pizza or pasta; it's a good source of magnesium, which helps relax blood vessels and muscles.

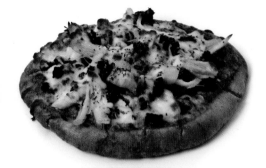

Perfect Pesto Pizza

Serves 4

4 (6") Sara Lee Mr. Pita Whole Wheat Pita Breads
8 Tbsp. DeLallo Pesto
1 tsp. salt and pepper
1 tsp. Italian seasoning
12 oz. fresh mozzarella, sliced
2 chicken breasts, cooked and shredded
¼ cup black olives, chopped
12 basil leaves, chopped
½ cup grated Parmesan

1. Preheat oven to 425° F. Warm pitas on a baking sheet in the oven for 5 minutes; remove.

2. Spread 2 Tbsp. of pesto sauce over each pita; top with mozzarella, chicken, olives, basil, Italian seasoning, salt, pepper, and Parmesan.

3. Bake for 8–10 minutes or until cheese is melted, and serve.

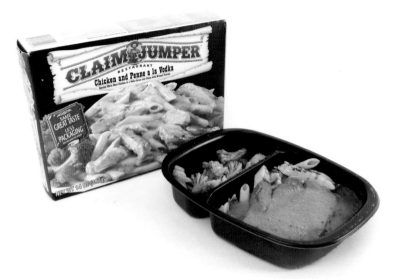

BELLY BAD

S/C Value = 8/3

Claim Jumper Chicken and Penne a la Vodka

Claim Jumper offers dense portions of food; this frozen version of one of their dishes is a smaller portion, but there's no shortage of sugar: 8 grams.

BELLY GOOD

S/C Value = 3/2

Chicken and Penne a la Vodka Do-Over:

Adding vodka to a sauce helps bring out the flavor in tomatoes. Only a small amount is added, and most of it burns off in the cooking process.

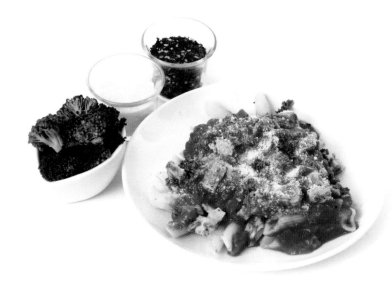

Delightful Penne Pasta

Serves 4

Pasta:
2 cups DeLallo Organic Whole Wheat Penne Rigate
1 cup Seeds of Change Vodka Americano Pasta
   Sauce
½ cup heavy cream
¼ cup chicken broth
½ tsp. red pepper flakes
½ Tbsp. salt and pepper
½ tsp. oregano
4 chicken breasts, cooked and diced
Chopped fresh Italian parsley, for garnish

Broccoli side:
2 cups broccoli florets
2 Tbsp. butter
2 Tbsp. Mrs. Dash Tomato Basil Garlic
   Seasoning Blend

Other sides:
¼ cup grated Parmesan
1 pinch red pepper flakes

1. For the pasta: Cook according to package directions; drain and set aside. In a saucepan, heat the pasta sauce, cream, chicken broth, and seasonings over medium heat until gently simmering. Add the chicken breasts and simmer for 5–7 minutes until chicken is heated through. Ladle the sauce over the pasta.

2. For the broccoli: Cook in a pot of boiling water for 2 minutes; drain. In the same pot, add the butter and seasoning over medium-high heat. When the butter has melted, add the broccoli and toss to coat. Remove from heat.

3. Dish out the pasta and sprinkle with Parmesan and red pepper flakes to taste. Garnish with chopped parsley and serve with cooked broccoli.

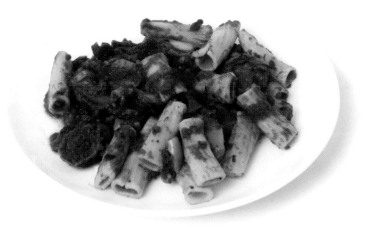

BELLY BAD

S/C Value = 6/3

BELLY GOOD

S/C Value = 2/2

Bertolli Italian Sausage & Rigatoni

Get rid of belly fat
and start feeling
healthy and energized
by keeping
your meals
at an S/C Value
of 5/2 or less.

Italian Sausage & Rigatoni Do-Over:

Arrabiata translates to
"angry dish," which is
perfect for this spicy
version of traditional pasta
sauce. Just add chili flakes
to taste if you want to
minimize the heat.

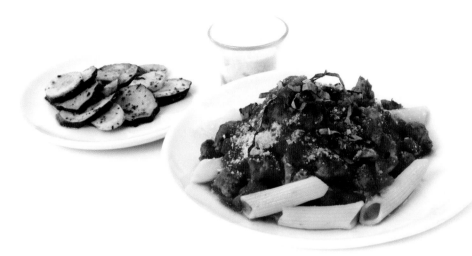

Spicy Sausage Pasta

Serves 4

Pasta:
2 cups DeLallo Organic Whole Wheat Penne
   Rigate, uncooked
1 cup Seeds of Change Marinara di Venezia
   Pasta Sauce
1 Tbsp. red pepper flakes (or more if desired)
¼ cup chicken broth
Salt and pepper to taste
2 cups cooked and crumbled Italian sausage
   (1 lb. uncooked)

Squash side:
¼ cup water
1 cup zucchini, sliced
1 cup yellow squash, sliced
Salt and pepper, to taste

Other side:
Grated Parmesan, to taste
¼ cup fresh basil leaves, chopped

1. For the pasta: Cook according to package directions; drain and set aside. In a saucepan, heat the sauce, broth, and red pepper flakes over medium heat until gently simmering. Add the sausage and let simmer for 5–7 minutes, until the sausage is heated through. Ladle the sauce over the pasta.

2. For the squash: Combine the water and squash in a pan; bring to a boil over medium heat. Cover and cook over low heat for 8–10 minutes or until tender. Drain, and season with salt and pepper to taste.

3. Dish out the pasta and sprinkle with Parmesan. Garnish with chopped basil and serve with cooked squash.

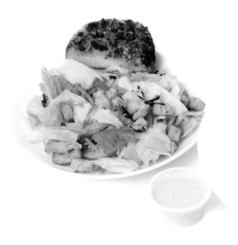

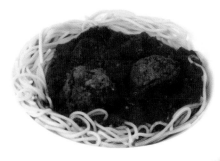

BELLY BAD

S/C Value = 24/9

Old Spaghetti Factory Spaghetti with Sicilian Meatballs

This traditional spaghetti and meatballs dinner covers almost 2 days on the Belly Fat Cure— in just 1 meal.

BELLY GOOD

S/C Value = 3/2

Spaghetti w/Meatballs Dinner Do-Over:

This Belly Fat Cure–approved meal will fulfill your pasta craving without filling out your waistline. Use bread from Ener-G Foods—there are only 7 grams of carbs per slice.

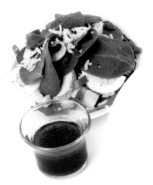
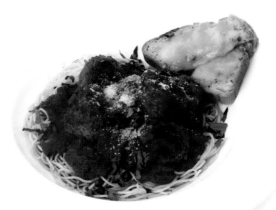

Tender Meatballs and Pasta

Serves 4

Pasta:
6 oz. De Cecco Whole Wheat Spaghetti, uncooked
1 cup Seeds of Change Tomato Basil Genovese
    Pasta Sauce
¼ cup chicken broth
12 Foster Farms Italian Style Turkey Meatballs,
    cooked
Grated Parmesan cheese for serving

Bread:
2 slices Ener-G Foods Light Brown Rice Loaf, cut in half
⅓ cup shredded Monterey Jack and cheddar cheese
    blend

Salad:
4 cups baby spinach leaves
1 hard-boiled egg, sliced
¼ cup shredded mozzarella
2 mushrooms, thinly sliced

Dressing:
⅓ cup extra-virgin olive oil
2 Tbsp. fresh lemon juice
Salt and pepper, to taste

1. For the pasta: Cook according to package directions; drain and set aside. In a medium saucepan, stir together the pasta sauce and broth over medium heat until simmering. Add meatballs and simmer until they're warmed through (approximately 10 minutes). Ladle the sauce over the pasta.

2. For the bread: Sprinkle the cheese over each half slice of bread and broil for 1–2 minutes or until cheese is melted.

3. For the salad: Arrange the spinach, eggs, mushrooms, and cheese on chilled salad plates.

4. For the dressing: Whisk together the olive oil and lemon juice; season with salt and pepper to taste. Dress the salads.

5. Dish out the pasta and sprinkle with Parmesan. Serve with bread and salad.

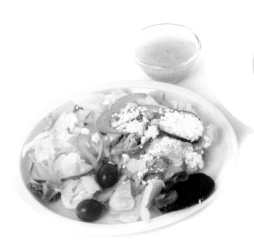

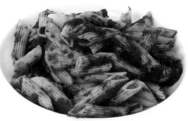

BELLY BAD

S/C Value = 24/6

BELLY GOOD

S/C Value = 4/2

Pat & Oscar's Pasta with Marinara & Greek Salad

This meal has 9 more grams of sugar than I recommend for an entire day! Make smarter choices every meal and you will lose belly fat.

Pasta with Marinara & Greek Salad Do-Over:

The sausage here is optional; you could go with no meat, or use chicken if you want a version that's lower in saturated fat.

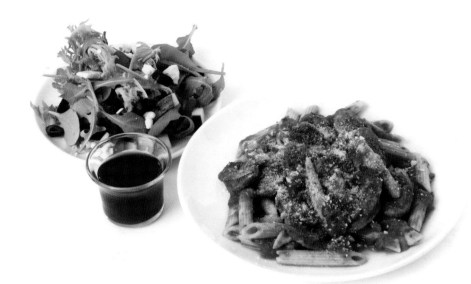

Tuscan Basil Penne

Serves 4

Pasta:
2 cups DeLallo Organic Whole Wheat Penne Rigate,
   uncooked
1 cup Seeds of Change Vodka Americano Pasta Sauce
¼ cup chicken broth
1 lb. Italian sausage, cooked and sliced
½ Tbsp. salt and pepper
¼ cup basil, chopped
Grated Parmesan

Salad:
1 (5 oz.) bag mixed salad greens
2 Tbsp. diced red onion
⅓ cup chopped cucumber
¼ cup chopped black olives
½ cup diced tomatoes
¼ cup crumbled feta cheese

Dressing:
⅓ cup extra-virgin olive oil
2 Tbsp. red-wine vinegar
Salt and pepper, to taste

1. For the pasta: Cook according to package directions; drain and set aside. In a saucepan, stir together the sauce and broth and heat over medium heat until gently simmering. Add cooked sausage and basil and simmer for 10 minutes. Ladle the sauce over the pasta.

2. For the salad: Toss together all salad ingredients and set aside.

3. For the dressing: Whisk together the olive oil and vinegar; season to taste with salt and pepper. Dress the salads.

4. Sprinkle the pasta with Parmesan to taste, and serve with salad.

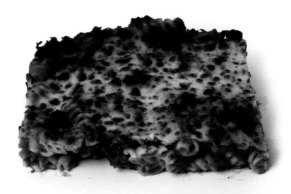

BELLY BAD

S/C Value = 10/3

BELLY GOOD

S/C Value = 1/2

Pizza Hut Meaty Marinara Baked Tuscani Pasta

Pizza Hut has beefed up their menu with a few pasta dishes. With a 10/3 S/C Value, this Meaty Marinara will also add some bulk to your belly.

Meaty Marinara Do-Over:

Be sure to check sugars and not just carbs on a pasta box—sometimes more than a couple grams sneak in.

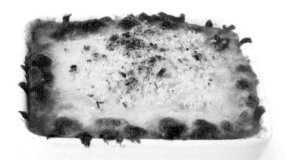

Rich and Meaty Pasta Bake

Serves 4

2 cups DeLallo Organic Whole Wheat
    Penne Rigate, uncooked
1 cup Seeds of Change Tomato Basil
    Genovese Pasta Sauce
¼ cup chicken broth
2 cups lean ground beef, cooked
Salt and pepper, to taste
¼ cup fresh basil, chopped
1 cup Jack and cheddar cheese, grated
¼ cup grated Parmesan cheese

1. Cook the pasta according to package directions;
drain and set aside. In a medium saucepan, heat
sauce and broth over medium heat until gently simmering. Add the cooked ground beef and let simmer
for 10 minutes; adjust seasoning with salt and pepper. Stir in the basil; remove from heat.

2. Mix the pasta with the meat sauce and divide
among 4 individual-size baking dishes. Top each
dish with grated Jack and cheddar cheese and a
sprinkle of Parmesan; broil until cheese is melted
and golden brown. Serve.

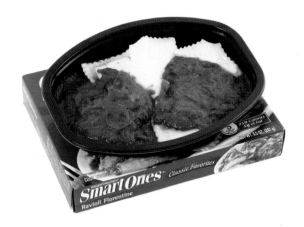

BELLY BAD

S/C Value = 12/2

BELLY GOOD

S/C Value = 2/2

Weight Watchers Smart Ones Ravioli Florentine

Frozen meals often have a long list of preservatives with names you don't understand; not only are they confusing, they can also add excessive amounts of sodium.

Ravioli Florentine Do-Over:

My ravioli dish is made with Rosetto All-Natural Whole Wheat Cheese Ravioli, which has 6 grams of fiber per serving—remember to select whole wheat whenever you can.

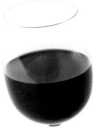

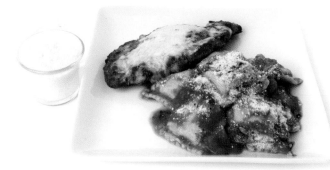

Ravioli Florentine

Serves 4

Ravioli:
2 cups Seeds of Change Marinara di Venezia
  Pasta Sauce
28 Rosetto All-Natural Whole Wheat Cheese
  Ravioli
2 Tbsp. extra-virgin olive oil
2 Tbsp. minced shallots
2 cloves garlic, minced
6 cups baby spinach leaves

Chicken:
4 chicken breasts
4 slices mozzarella

Other sides:
1 (5 oz. serving) glass red wine per person
¼ cup grated Parmesan cheese

1. For the ravioli: Cook according to package directions; drain and set aside. In a large skillet, heat 1 Tbsp. of the olive oil over medium heat. Sauté shallots and garlic until brown, and sauté spinach until wilted. Add the pasta sauce and simmer for 10 minutes.

2. For the chicken: Preheat oven to 350° F. Heat a large skillet over medium-high heat; add the remaining Tbsp. of olive oil. Add the breasts and cook 4 minutes per side. Transfer to a large baking dish; bake 8–10 minutes or until cooked through. Top each breast with a slice of cheese. Return to the oven and cook until the cheese melts and is bubbly, about 2–4 minutes.

3. Divide the ravioli into 4 servings and top each of them with ½ cup of the sauce. Serve with a mozzarella-topped chicken breast and a sprinkling of Parmesan. Enjoy with a glass of red wine.

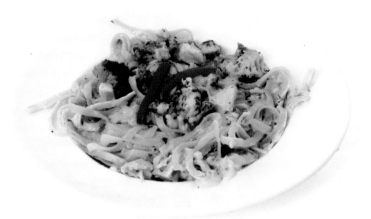

BELLY BAD

S/C Value = 10/6

Uno Chicago Grill Chicken, Broccoli & Fettuccine

We don't track calories on the Belly Fat Cure, but it's important to note that this dish has 1,300 calories . . . along with more than 2,000 milligrams of sodium.

BELLY GOOD

S/C Value = 4/2

Chicken Fettuccine Alfredo Do-Over:

I recommend Kirkland Signature Seasoned Rotisserie Chickens—they are tasty and cut out cooking time. But you can also make this meal without meat if you'd like.

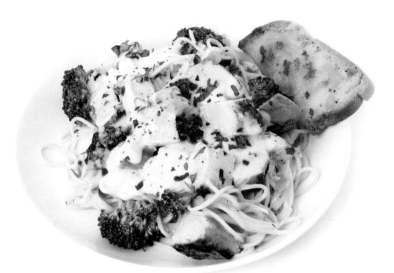

Creamy Chicken Alfredo Pasta

Serves 4

Pasta:

6 oz. De Cecco Whole Wheat Spaghetti,
   uncooked
½ cup Classico Creamy Alfredo Sauce
½ cup chicken broth
1 cup broccoli florets, chopped
2 chicken breasts, cooked and diced
¼ cup basil, chopped
2 Tbsp. oregano, chopped
¼ cup grated Parmesan
¼ cup parsley, chopped

Cheesy bread:

2 slices Ener-G Foods Light Brown Rice Loaf
⅓ cup shredded Monterey Jack and cheddar
   cheese blend

1. For the pasta: Cook according to package directions; drain and set aside. In a medium saucepan, stir together the sauce and broth over medium heat until simmering. Add the chicken and cook until warmed through (approximately 5–7 minutes). Add the broccoli and cook for 2–3 minutes more. Add the sauce to the pasta.

2. For the bread: Cut each piece in half and place the cheese on top. Broil for 1–2 minutes or until the cheese is melted.

3. Toss the pasta with basil, oregano, and Parmesan. Garnish with parsley, add a slice of cheesy bread, and serve.

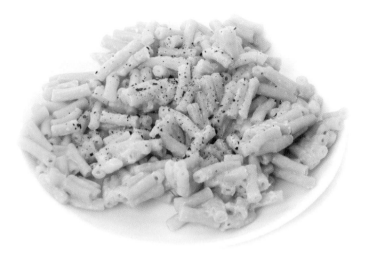

BELLY BAD

S/C Value = 10/3

Mimi's Café Kraft Macaroni and Cheese

This mac 'n' cheese dish off the kids' menu at Mimi's Café looks just like the popular box version, except Kraft's has less sugar (although it's still too much).

BELLY GOOD

S/C Value = 2/2

Macaroni and Cheese Do-Over:

Just about everyone will agree that macaroni and cheese is one of their favorite comfort foods. The bread crumbs give this one a little crunchy kick.

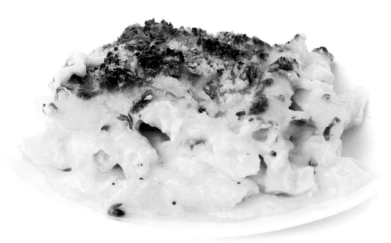

Extraordinary Mac 'n' Cheese

Serves 4

2 cups DeLallo Organic Whole Wheat Penne
  Rigate
6 Tbsp. unsalted butter, divided use
3 Tbsp. Arrowhead Mills Organic Soy Flour
2 cups heavy cream
2½ cups shredded extra-sharp cheddar cheese,
  divided use
¾ cup grated Parmesan cheese, divided use
2 tsp. Lawry's Seasoned Salt
Reserved pasta water
2 Tbsp. panko (Japanese bread crumbs)
1 Tbsp. finely chopped parsley, for garnish

1. For the pasta: Preheat oven to 400° F and place
the rack in the middle of the oven. Prepare pasta
according to package directions; drain (save some
pasta water in case the sauce is too thick) and set
aside. Melt 4 Tbsp. of butter in a large saucepan

over medium-low heat; stir in flour constantly for 3
minutes. Whisk in cream and bring the sauce to a
boil while still whisking. Reduce heat to medium low,
whisking for another 3 minutes. Stir in 2 cups of the
cheddar, half of the Parmesan, and the seasoning
until smooth (add reserved pasta water if the sauce
is too thick). Remove from heat, stir in the cooked
pasta, and transfer to a baking dish.

2. For the topping: Melt the remaining 2 Tbsp. of
butter; stir together with the panko and remaining
cheeses in a bowl until combined well. Sprinkle over
the pasta and place it all in the preheated oven for
15–20 minutes, until bubbling and golden brown.
Remove.

3. Garnish with parsley and serve.

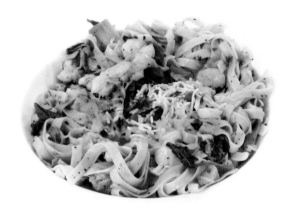

BELLY BAD

S/C Value = 24/6

Mimi's Café Mediterranean Chicken Fettuccine

This mostly colorless dish doesn't have a lot of nutritional value. It's best to try to eat fruits and vegetables of different colors every day in order

BELLY GOOD

S/C Value = 3/2

Mediterranean Chicken Fettuccine Do-Over:

Venture away from the Parmesan that comes in a green can and try grating it fresh instead. You'll be amazed at the flavor—a little goes a long way!

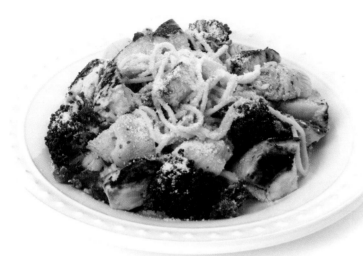

Chicken Parmesan Pasta

Serves 4

6 oz. De Cecco Whole Wheat Spaghetti,
    uncooked
4 Tbsp. butter
2 shallots, chopped
2 garlic cloves, minced
12 oz. precooked chicken strips
2 cups broccoli florets
3 artichoke hearts, chopped
2 Tbsp. sun-dried tomatoes
¼ cup chopped basil
½ cup chicken broth
½ cup grated Parmesan, plus more
    for serving

1. Prepare pasta according to package instructions; drain and set aside. Melt the butter in a large skillet on medium-high heat. Sauté the shallots and garlic until brown. Add the chicken, broccoli, artichoke hearts, sun-dried tomatoes, and basil. Add the chicken broth and bring to a boil; reduce the heat and simmer for 10 minutes. Add the Parmesan cheese to achieve desired thickness of the sauce, stirring in cheese as it melts. Remove from heat.

2. Combine the sauce and pasta and transfer to a baking dish. Put it in the oven for 15–20 minutes, until bubbling and golden brown; remove.

3. Serve hot with additional Parmesan on the side.

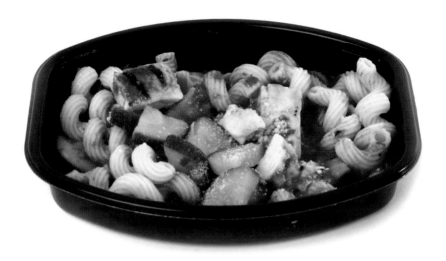

BELLY BAD

S/C Value = 10/2

Lean Cuisine Sun-Dried Tomato Pesto Chicken

This dish knocks out more than half of your sugar grams for the day. Check out the food list in Chapter 6 for other Lean Cuisine dishes that are Belly Fat Cure–approved.

BELLY GOOD

S/C Value = 5/2

Sun-Dried Tomato Pesto Do-Over:

Zucchini is an excellent source of manganese, a trace mineral that helps stimulate important enzymes in your body. You could try this dish with yellow squash, too.

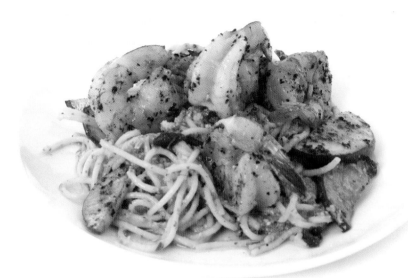

Succulent Shrimp & Pesto Pasta

Serves 4

6 oz. De Cecco Whole Wheat Spaghetti,
  uncooked
½ cup DeLallo Pesto
½ cup chicken broth
2 Tbsp. extra-virgin olive oil
½ lb. medium shrimp, peeled and uncooked
1 Tbsp. Lawry's Seasoned Salt
⅓ cup sun-dried tomatoes
1 cup sliced zucchini
½ cup grated Parmesan
½ cup chopped basil

1. For the pasta: Prepare according to package
instructions; drain and set aside.

2. For the shrimp: Heat the olive oil in a medium
skillet over medium heat until it begins to shim-
mer. Add the shrimp and sauté until they become
opaque (approximately 3–5 minutes). Add the
pesto sauce and broth and bring to a simmer.
Stir in the seasoning, sun-dried tomatoes, and
zucchini. Cook for 3 minutes and pour over
pasta. Top with basil and Parmesan and serve.

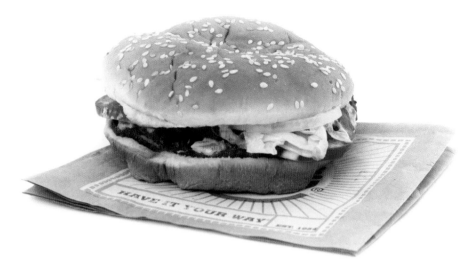

BELLY BAD

S/C Value = 11/3

BELLY GOOD

S/C Value = 1/2

Burger King Whopper with Cheese

The Whopper's been around since 1957; if you eat this burger with its 11 grams of sugar, your belly fat's going to stick around just as long.

Whopper with Cheese Do-Over:

If you're grill-less or it's winter, try out a grill pan, which gives the same effect (lines and all) without having to leave the stove.

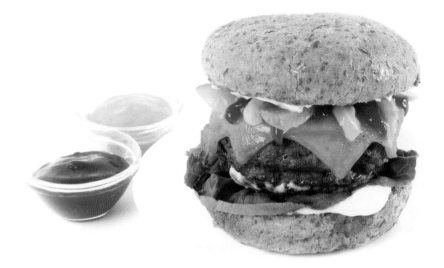

Melted Cheddar Cheeseburger

Serves 4

1¼ lbs. lean ground beef
Salt and pepper, to taste
8 slices cheddar cheese
4 Food for Life Ezekiel 4:9 Sprouted Grain
    Burger Buns
8 dill pickle slices
4 romaine lettuce leaves
4 Tbsp. mayonnaise
4 Tbsp. mustard
2 Tbsp. Nature's Hollow Sugar Free Ketchup

1. Preheat grill to medium-high heat. Divide meat and form into 4 patties; season as desired. When the grill is ready, cook each burger about 4–6 minutes per side. Top each patty with 2 cheese slices; close the grill and cook for 1 more minute or until the cheese starts to melt.

2. Build the burgers to your liking using dill pickles, lettuce, mayonnaise, mustard, and ketchup. Enjoy!

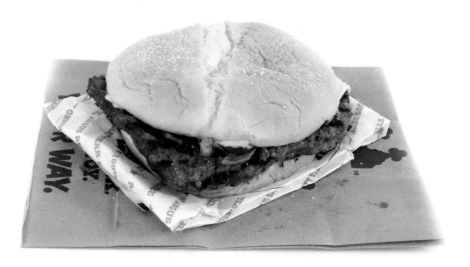

BELLY BAD

S/C Value = 11/3

BELLY GOOD

S/C Value = 1/2

Burger King Mushroom Swiss Steakhouse XT Burger

Perhaps it's the mysterious sauce on this burger that gives it almost a whole day's worth of sugar. It also takes half of your carbs for the day, without any whole-grain benefits.

Mushroom Swiss Steakhouse Burger Do-Over:

One Food for Life Ezekiel 4:9 Sprouted Grain Burger Bun has 6 grams of dietary fiber—eating 25–30 grams of fiber a day will help ensure that you lose false belly fat.

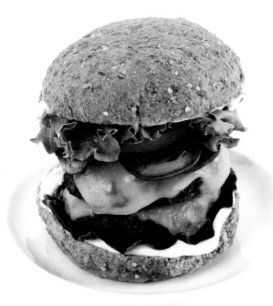

Simple Swiss & Mushroom Burger

Serves 4

2 Tbsp. extra-virgin olive oil
1 cup mushrooms, sliced
3 cloves garlic, chopped
2 lbs. lean ground beef
Salt and pepper, to taste
8 slices Swiss cheese
4 Food for Life Ezekiel 4:9 Sprouted Grain
    Burger Buns
4 red-leaf lettuce leaves
4 thin slices of tomato
4 Tbsp. mayonnaise
4 Tbsp. mustard

1. Preheat grill to medium to high heat. Heat the olive oil in a skillet on medium high. Sauté the mushrooms and garlic until the water released from the mushrooms has evaporated; set aside. Divide meat and form into 8 patties; season as desired. When the grill is ready, cook each burger about 4–6 minutes per side. Divide mushrooms onto each burger and place 1 slice of Swiss cheese on top; close the grill and cook for 1 more minute or until the cheese starts to melt.

2. Build these double burgers to your liking using lettuce, tomato slices, mayonnaise, and mustard. Enjoy!

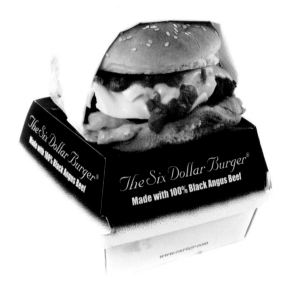

BELLY BAD

S/C Value = 10/3

Carl's Jr. Guacamole Bacon Six Dollar Burger

The hamburger bun could be the main culprit in this burger, giving it 10 grams of sugar. Be sure to check the sugar content of all your favorite breads and buns.

BELLY GOOD

S/C Value = 1/2

Guacamole Bacon Burger Do-Over:

Avocados contain a monounsaturated fat called oleic acid that's shown to help lower cholesterol. Mix them with a few simple ingredients for great-tasting guacamole.

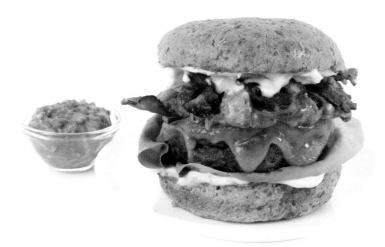

Decadent Guacamole Burger

Serves 4

Guacamole:

1 cup mashed avocado

3 Tbsp. diced tomato

3 Tbsp. diced onion

¼ cup chopped fresh cilantro

Juice from ½ a lime

Salt and pepper, to taste

Burger:

1¼ lbs. lean ground beef

4 slices cheddar cheese

4 Food for Life Ezekiel 4:9 Sprouted Grain
   Burger Buns

8 strips of bacon, cooked, each slice cut in half

4 Tbsp. mayonnaise

4 leaves Bibb (or Boston or butter leaf) lettuce

1. For the guacamole: Mix together the mashed avocado, tomato, onion, cilantro, and lime juice. Season to taste.

2. For the burgers: Preheat grill to medium-high heat. Divide meat and form into 4 patties; season to taste. When the grill is ready, cook each burger about 4–6 minutes per side. Top each patty with 1 slice of cheese; grill for 1 more minute or until the cheese starts to melt.

3. Build the burgers to your liking using bacon, mayonnaise, lettuce—and don't forget the guaca-mole! Olé!

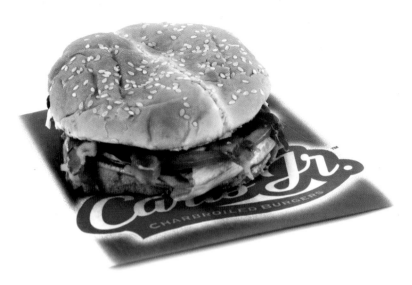

BELLY BAD

S/C Value = 24/4

BELLY GOOD

S/C Value = 2/2

Carl's Jr./Hardee's Kentucky Bourbon Burger

With nearly two days' worth of sugar, this burger will bulk up your belly in no time. The bourbon sauce could add more than 15 grams of sugar on its own.

Kentucky Bourbon Burger Do-Over:

Is it possible to make a barbecue burger with 1 gram of sugar? Yes! We used Scott's Barbecue Sauce, which is both sugar and fat free, yet full of spice and flavor.

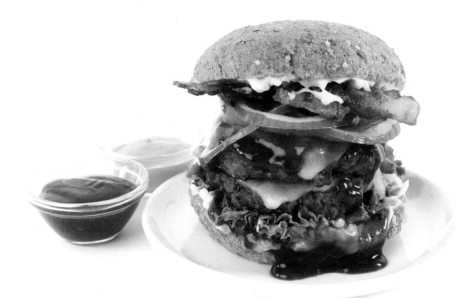

Wild-West Bacon Burger

Serves 4

2 lbs. lean ground beef
Salt and pepper, to taste
8 slices pepper Jack cheese
4 Food for Life Ezekiel 4:9 Sprouted Grain
    Burger Buns
8 strips of bacon, cooked, each slice cut in half
4 romaine lettuce leaves
4 thin slices of red onion
4 thin slices of tomato
4 Tbsp. mayonnaise
2 Tbsp. mustard
8 Tbsp. Scott's Barbecue Sauce

1. Preheat grill to medium-high heat. Divide meat and form into 8 patties; season to taste. When the grill is ready, cook each burger about 4–6 minutes per side. Top each patty with 1 slice of cheese; close the grill for 1 more minute or until the cheese starts to melt.

2. Build these double burgers to your liking using bacon, lettuce, onion, tomato, mayonnaise, mustard—and, of course, barbecue sauce! Round 'em up!

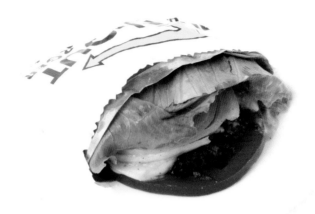

BELLY BAD

S/C Value = 7/1

In-N-Out
Double Double Protein
Style Burger

In-N-Out almost gets it
right. But if you want to
lose belly fat, 7 grams
of sugar is still too
many for one meal;
remember, stick to
5 or fewer.

BELLY GOOD

S/C Value = 2/1

Protein Style
Burger
Do-Over:

When you want the
lighter version of a tasty
double cheeseburger,
try this one, which uses
lettuce instead of a bun.
Top with Nature's Hollow
Sugar Free Ketchup.

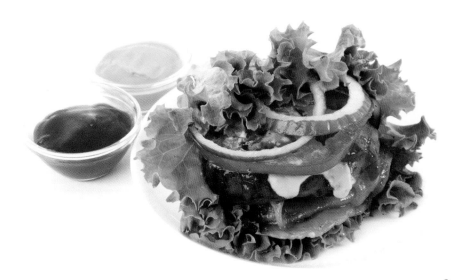

Lighter Side Cheesy Burger

Serves 4

2 lbs. lean ground beef
2 eggs, beaten
1 Tbsp. minced garlic
½ cup finely chopped onion
Salt and pepper to taste
8 slices cheddar cheese
2 Tbsp. mustard
2 Tbsp. Nature's Hollow Sugar Free Ketchup
4 thin slices of tomato
4 thin slices of red onion
8 leaves green-leaf lettuce

1. Preheat grill to medium-high heat. Thoroughly combine the first 4 ingredients. Divide meat and form into 8 patties; season to taste. When the grill is ready, cook each burger about 4–6 minutes per side. Top each patty with a slice of cheese; close the grill and cook for 1 more minute or until the cheese starts to melt.

2. Stack two burgers and spread with ketchup and mustard, then top with tomato and onion slices. Wrap between two leaves of lettuce and serve.

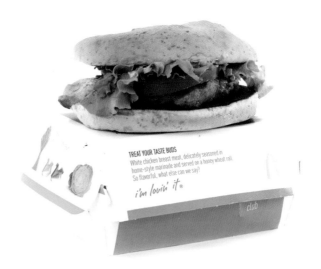

TREAT YOUR TASTE BUDS
White chicken breast meat, delicately seasoned in home-style marinade and served on a honey wheat roll. So flavorful, what else can we say?

i'm lovin' it®

club

BELLY BAD

S/C Value = 11/3

BELLY GOOD

S/C Value = 0/2

McDonald's Premium Grilled Chicken Classic Sandwich

Nearly all of McDonald's sandwiches have more than 5 grams of sugar—where'd they hide it? Blame the bun.

Chicken Classic Sandwich Do-Over:

You can add barbecue sauce to this recipe if you wish. Just be sure to use Scott's, which is sugar free and can be used on poultry, meat, fish, and seafood.

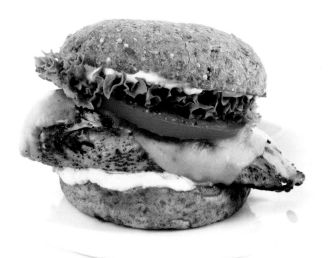

Classic Chicken Burger

Serves 4

4 chicken breasts
Salt and pepper, to taste
4 slices Monterey Jack cheese
4 Food for Life Ezekiel 4:9 Sprouted
    Grain Burger Buns
4 leaves or green-leaf or butter lettuce
4 thin slices of tomato
4 Tbsp. mayonnaise

1. Preheat grill to medium to high heat. When the grill is ready, season the chicken breasts to taste and cook until done, approximately 5–7 minutes per side. Top each breast with a slice of cheese; close the grill and cook for 1 more minute or until the cheese starts to melt.

2. Build the sandwiches to your liking using lettuce, tomato, and mayonnaise.

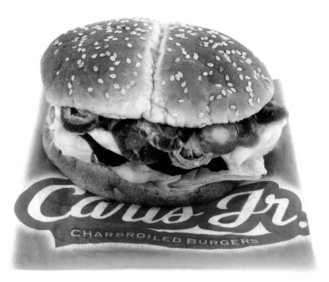

BELLY BAD

S/C Value = 9/3

BELLY GOOD

S/C Value = 2/2

Carl's Jr. Jalapeño Burger

You can get spicy without the sugar by making smarter choices. Skip this version from Carl's Jr.; 9 grams in one meal will help you gain, not lose, belly fat.

Jalapeño Burger Do-Over:

I mixed Serrano chilies in with the ground beef to give this burger a little extra kick. And note that chipotles are smoked jalapeños with mild heat.

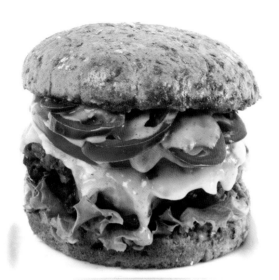

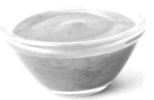

Super Spicy Burger

Serves 4

Burger:

1¼ lb. lean ground beef

1 egg, beaten

2 garlic cloves, finely chopped

2–3 Serrano chilies, finely chopped

2 Tbsp. Dijon mustard

2 tsp. chili powder

8 slices Monterey Jack or pepper Jack cheese

4 Food for Life Ezekiel 4:9 Sprouted Grain
　Burger Buns

4 large green-leaf lettuce leaves

4 thin slices of tomato

4 thin rings of green bell pepper

Chipotle sauce:

2 tsp. chipotle pepper in adobo sauce, minced

¼ cup mayonnaise

2 Tbsp. sour cream

1. For the burgers: Preheat grill to medium to high heat. Thoroughly combine the first 6 ingredients in a bowl. Divide and form into 4 patties. When the grill is ready, cook each burger about 4–6 minutes per side. Top each patty with a slice of cheese; close the grill and cook for 1 more minute or until the cheese starts to melt.

2. For the sauce: Mix the chipotle pepper, mayonnaise, and sour cream together.

3. Build the burgers to your liking, using lettuce, tomato, bell pepper—and, of course, chipotle sauce! Kick it up!

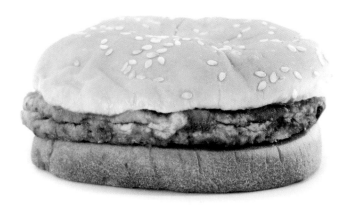

BELLY BAD

S/C Value = 8/3

BELLY GOOD

S/C Value = 1/2

Burger King BK Veggie Burger

Veggie doesn't always mean healthy. This burger, for instance, has more than half the amount of sugar you should have in one day. See the food list in Chapter 6 for smarter options.

Veggie Burger Do-Over:

By using Morningstar Farms Grillers Prime patties, we can make this veggie burger with no sugar. Add cheese if you'd like— it's a 0/0.

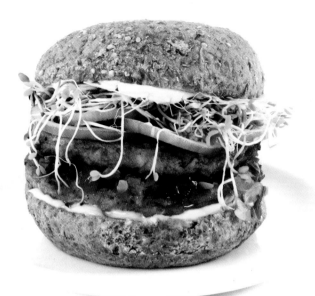

Very Veggie Burger

Serves 4

4 Morningstar Farms Grillers Prime
    Veggie Burgers
4 Tbsp. mayonnaise
4 Tbsp. Dijon mustard
4 Food for Life Ezekiel 4:9 Sprouted
    Grain Burger Buns
1 cup alfalfa sprouts
4 thin slices of red onion
4 Tbsp. Heinz Dill Relish

1. Preheat grill to medium to high heat (veggie burgers can be made in the microwave, but a grill is recommended). When the grill is ready, cook each patty about 3 minutes or until middle is cooked through.

2. In a small bowl, stir together the mayonnaise and Dijon mustard. Spread the mixture on the buns, and build the burgers using sprouts, onions, and relish.

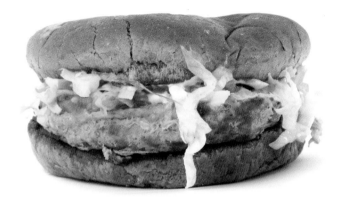

BELLY BAD

S/C Value = 10/3

Fatburger
Turkey Burger

Lower in fat than Fatburger's beef burger, this sandwich has more sugar—double what you should eat in one meal. Have a hot dog instead if you stop here.

BELLY GOOD

S/C Value = 1/2

Turkey Burger
Do-Over:

Adding garlic to this turkey burger gives it a boost of the antioxidant vitamin C. Garlic also helps relax your blood vessels—a heart-healthy benefit.

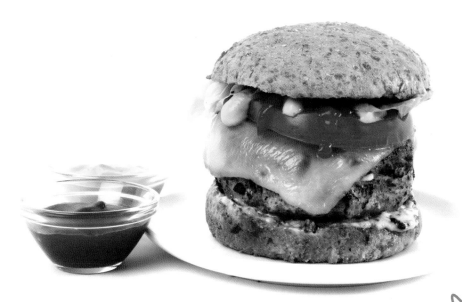

Ultimate Turkey Burger

Serves 4

1¼ lb. ground turkey
2 cloves garlic, chopped
1½ Tbsp. low-sodium soy sauce
1 green onion, chopped
4 slices Monterey Jack cheese
4 Food for Life Ezekiel 4:9 Sprouted Grain
    Burger Buns
4 green-leaf lettuce leaves
4 thin slices tomato
4 Tbsp. mayonnaise
2 Tbsp. Nature's Hollow Sugar Free Ketchup
4 Tbsp. mustard

1. Preheat grill to medium to high heat. Thoroughly combine the first 4 ingredients in a bowl; divide and form into 4 patties. When the grill is ready, cook each burger about 5 minutes per side. Top each patty with a slice of cheese; close the grill, and cook for 1 more minute or until the cheese starts to melt.

2. Build the burgers to your liking using lettuce, tomato, and condiments. Enjoy!

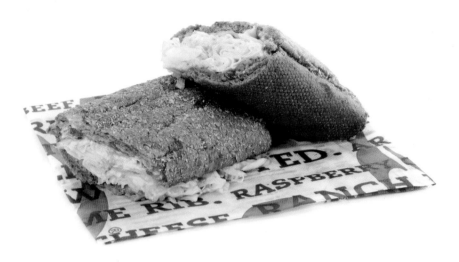

BELLY BAD

S/C Value = 8/4

Quiznos Turkey Ranch & Swiss

With 74 grams of carbs, this single sandwich eats up more than half of your entire carb allotment for the day—and that's just the regular size. A large has *102* grams!

BELLY GOOD

S/C Value = 0/2

Turkey Ranch & Swiss Do-Over:

Look for antibiotic-free sliced turkey that has no nitrates, which are preservatives that convert into a cancer-promoting carcinogen.

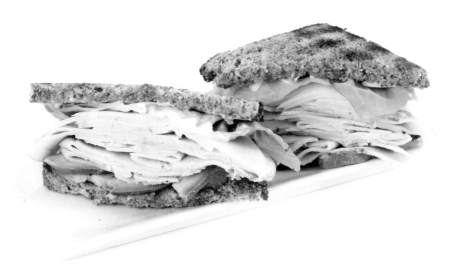

Smokey Turkey Sandwich

Serves 4

8 slices Food for Life Ezekiel 4:9 Sprouted 100% Whole Grain Bread (toasted if desired)
4 Tbsp. Dijon mustard
4 Tbsp. mayonnaise
12 oz. sliced smoked turkey
4 slices provolone
4 leaves Bibb (or Boston or butter leaf) lettuce
1 avocado, sliced

1. Using 2 slices of bread per sandwich, spread mustard and mayonnaise on each slice. Build each sandwich by stacking the bottom slice of bread with avocado, sliced turkey, provolone, lettuce, and the top slice of bread. Serve.

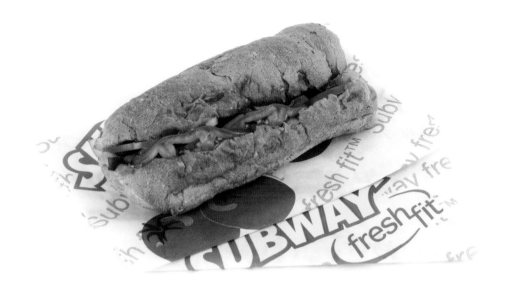

BELLY BAD

S/C Value = 10/3

BELLY GOOD

S/C Value = 3/2

Subway 6" Sweet Onion Chicken Teriyaki Sandwich

A few Subway sandwiches have an S/C Value of 5/2 or less, but not this one. Don't be fooled by "fat free" Sweet Onion Sauce—it has 8 grams of sugar.

Sweet Onion Chicken Teriyaki Sandwich Do-Over:

Watch for the label on Oroweat products that says: "No High-Fructose Corn Syrup." Note that the company has stopped using HFCS in its products.

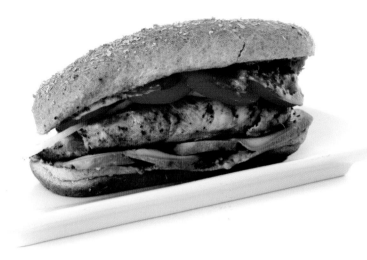

Spicy Dijon Chicken Sandwich

Serves 4

4 large chicken breasts, grilled
Salt and black pepper or Lawry's
    Lemon Pepper, to taste
4 Tbsp. Dijon mustard
4 Tbsp. mayonnaise
1 avocado, sliced
8 thin slices of tomato
8 slices Monterey Jack cheese
4 Oroweat 100% Whole Wheat
    Hot Dog Buns

1. Preheat grill to medium heat. Season chicken with salt and pepper. When the grill is ready, cook the chicken breasts until done, approximately 5–7 minutes per side.

2. Toast the buns on the grill, if desired. Spread buns with mustard and mayonnaise. Build each sandwich with avocado, chicken, cheese, and tomato. Serve.

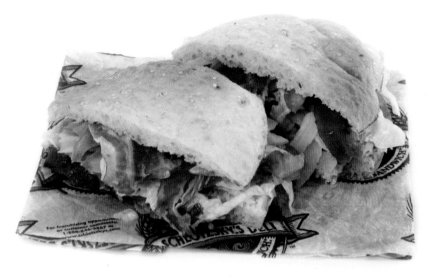

BELLY BAD

S/C Value = 5/4

BELLY GOOD

S/C Value = 1/2

Schlotzsky's BLT

While this BLT just makes it on the sugar mark, 74 grams of carbs gives it a 4 on the S/C Value. This isn't the worst on our list, but you can make a smarter choice.

BLT Do-Over:

I'm using Food for Life Ezekiel 4:9 bread here—with just 15 grams of carbs and no sugar, it makes a smarter sandwich simple.

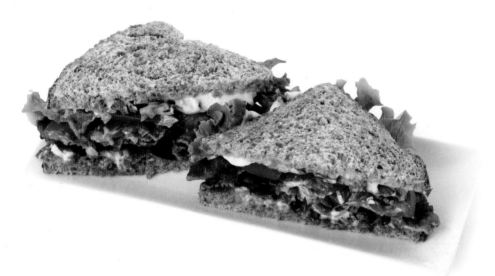

Old-School BLT

Serves 4

8 slices Food for Life Ezekiel 4:9 Sprouted 100% Whole Grain Bread
4 Tbsp. mayonnaise
12 strips of bacon, cooked, each slice cut in half
8 thin slices of tomato
1 tsp. Lawry's Seasoned Pepper or Lemon Pepper
8 leaves Bibb (or Boston or butter leaf) lettuce

1. Toast the bread. Lay out 2 slices per sandwich and spread mustard and mayonnaise on each slice. Build sandwiches by stacking the bottom slice of bread with bacon, tomatoes, seasoning, lettuce, and the top slice of bread. Serve.

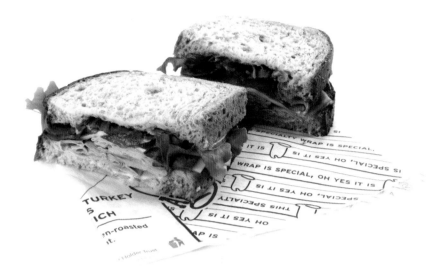

BELLY BAD

S/C Value = 19/4

BELLY GOOD

S/C Value = 2/2

Arby's Roast Ham & Swiss Sandwich

This sandwich looks innocent, but it has 19 grams of belly fat–promoting sugar— that's almost 5 tsp. of sugar and more than you should have in an entire day.

Roast Ham & Swiss Sandwich Do-Over:

Look for organic tomatoes for your sandwiches— research has shown that they have higher levels of *flavonoids,* which are compounds that help protect against cardio-vascular disease.

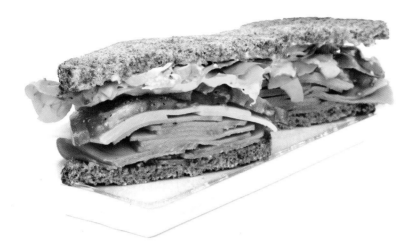

Ham & Cheese Sandwich

Serves 4

8 slices Food for Life Ezekiel 4:9 Sprouted
    100% Whole Grain Bread
4 Tbsp. mustard
2 Tbsp. mayonnaise
1½ lbs. sliced ham
8 slices Jarlsberg or Emmenthaler cheese
8 thin slices of tomato
1 tsp. Lawry's Seasoned Pepper or Lemon
    Pepper
8 butter lettuce leaves

1. Lay out 2 slices of bread and spread mustard and mayonnaise on each slice. Build sandwiches by stacking the bottom slice of bread with ham, cheese, tomatoes, seasoning, lettuce, and the top slice of bread. Serve.

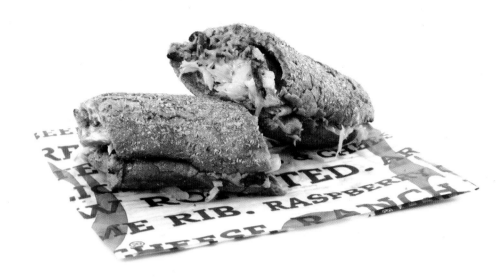

BELLY BAD

S/C Value = 9/4

BELLY GOOD

S/C Value = 2/2

Quiznos Roast Beef & Cheddar

On top of the
9/4 S/C Value,
this sandwich has
more than 2,100 milligrams
of sodium—as much
as you should have
in an entire day.

Roast Beef & Cheddar Do-Over:

A little rosemary adds a
fresh taste and surprising
health benefits—the aro-
matic pine-like herb aids
in digestion and immune
health and improves
circulation.

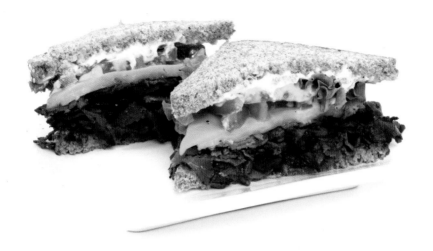

Beef & Cheddar Sandwich

Serves 4

2 Tbsp. red-wine vinegar
2 Tbsp. extra-virgin olive oil
1 tsp. fresh rosemary, very finely chopped
8 slices Food for Life Ezekiel 4:9 Sprouted
    100% Whole Grain Bread
4 Tbsp. mustard
4 Tbsp. mayonnaise
1½ lbs. deli-sliced roast beef
8 slices cheddar cheese
8 thin slices of tomato
1 pinch Lawry's Lemon Pepper
4 romaine lettuce leaves

1. Mix the first 3 ingredients in a bottle with a lid and shake (or whisk in a bowl); set aside.

2. Lay out 2 slices of bread per sandwich and spread mustard and mayonnaise on each slice. Build sandwiches by stacking the bottom slice of bread with roast beef and drizzling on a little of the rosemary dressing; add 2 slices of cheese and tomato, seasoning, lettuce, and another drizzle of rosemary dressing. Finish with the top slice of bread and serve.

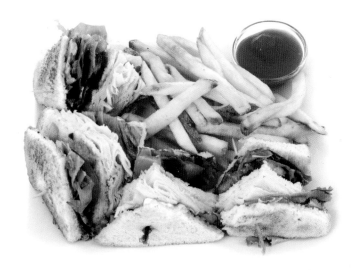

BELLY BAD

S/C Value = 17/6

Denny's Club Sandwich

With 119 grams of carbs, this dish does away with your allotment for the entire day. The only sandwich on the Denny's menu that comes close to being Belly Fat Cure–approved is The Super Bird sandwich, with a 3/3 S/C Value.

BELLY GOOD

S/C Value = 5/2

Club Sandwich Do-Over:

We used Oroweat Light 100% Whole Wheat Bread here. With only 9 carb grams, this bread allows you to enjoy a traditional club with three slices of bread.

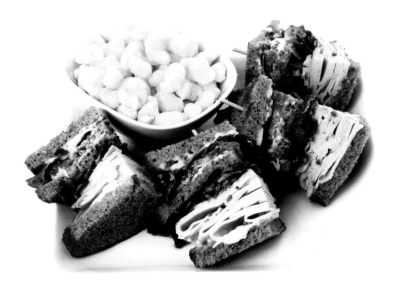

Distinctive Club Sandwich

Serves 4

Sandwich:

12 slices Oroweat Light 100% Whole
   Wheat Bread

4 Tbsp. mayonnaise

12 oz. smoked turkey

12 strips of bacon, cooked and cut in half

4 thin slices of tomato

1 tsp. Lawry's Seasoned Pepper or Lemon
   Pepper

8 Bibb (or Boston or butter leaf) lettuce leaves

Other sides:

2 oz. Pirate's Booty Aged White Cheddar Snack

1. Toast the bread. Lay out 3 slices per sandwich, and spread mayonnaise on each slice. Build sandwiches by stacking the bottom slice of bread with turkey and bacon, the middle slice of bread, tomatoes, seasoning, lettuce, and the top slice of bread. Serve.

2. Serve each sandwich with equal amounts of Pirate's Booty.

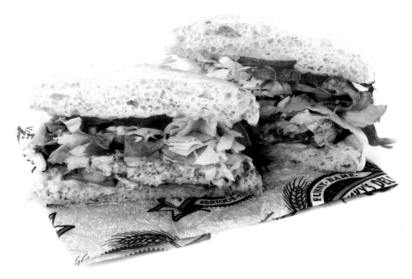

BELLY BAD

S/C Value = 4/4

BELLY GOOD

S/C Value = 1/2

Schlotzsky's Homestyle Tuna Sandwich

While this sandwich isn't as bad as what you'd find at Schlotzsky's sister companies, Carvel and Cinnabon, its 4/4 S/C Value isn't exactly ideal for losing belly fat.

Tuna Sandwich Do-Over:

Add eggs for a little extra protein and choline, a type of B vitamin that helps keep cell membranes healthy and reduces inflammation.

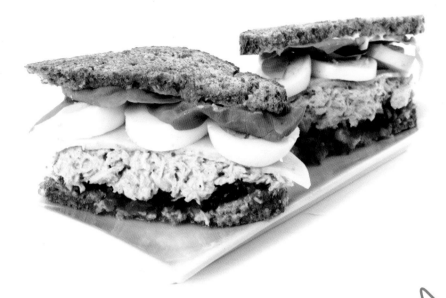

Tempting Tuna Sandwich

Serves 4

2 (6 oz.) cans of solid white tuna in water, drained
4 Tbsp. mayonnaise
2 Tbsp. Dijon mustard
2 Tbsp. Heinz Dill Relish
2 tsp. onion powder
Salt and pepper, to taste
8 slices Food for Life Ezekiel 4:9 Sprouted 100% Whole Grain Bread
4 slices cheese of your choice
2 hard-boiled eggs, sliced
1 cup spinach

1. Thoroughly combine the first 6 ingredients in a bowl.

2. Lay out 2 slices of bread per sandwich. Build sandwiches by spreading the tuna mixture over the bottom slice of bread, then layering with cheese, sliced egg, spinach, and the top slice of bread. Serve.

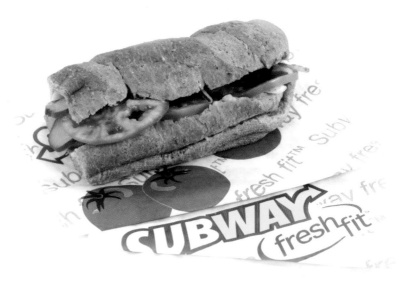

BELLY BAD

S/C Value = 7/3

BELLY GOOD

S/C Value = 3/2

Subway 6"
Veggie Delite Sandwich

Even though this sandwich
is promoted as "low fat,"
it's high enough in
sugar and carbs to
get in the way of
your belly fat loss.

Veggie Delite
Sandwich Do-Over:

Portobello mushrooms
are a good source of
potassium and selenium,
a trace mineral that's been
shown to reduce the risk
of prostate cancer.

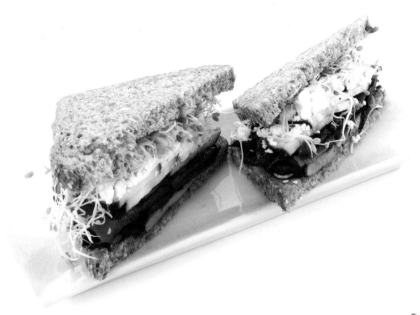

Fresh Veggie Sandwich

Serves 4

2 Tbsp. butter
1 portobello mushroom, sliced
2 Tbsp. red-wine vinegar
2 Tbsp. extra-virgin olive oil
4 Tbsp. Dijon mustard
½ cup fresh basil, chopped
8 slices Food for Life Ezekiel 4:9 Sprouted
    100% Whole Grain Bread
⅓ cup roasted red peppers, sliced
1 cup sliced cucumber
2 cups alfalfa sprouts
1 cup feta cheese

1. In a large skillet over medium-high heat, melt the butter. When the butter has melted, sauté the mushrooms until golden; set aside to cool. Add the vinegar, oil, mustard, and chopped basil to a blender and puree until smooth; transfer to a small bowl.

2. Lay out 2 slices of bread per sandwich, and spread the basil-mustard mixture on each slice. Build sandwiches by layering the bottom slice of bread with mushrooms, red peppers, sliced cucumbers, sprouts, and feta. Add the top slice of bread and serve.

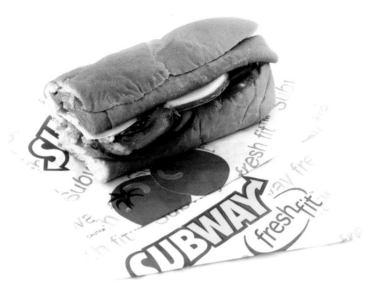

BELLY BAD

S/C Value = 8/3

Subway 6"
Cold Cut Combo

Surprisingly, a tuna sandwich at Subway has more fat than this Italian favorite. Of course, 8 grams of sugar will still make losing belly fat difficult; stick with 5/2 or under per meal.

BELLY GOOD

S/C Value = 4/2

Cold Cut Combo
Do-Over:

Enjoy these subs on Oroweat 100% Whole Wheat Hot Dog Buns—they have 28 carb grams per bun and 6 grams of fiber.

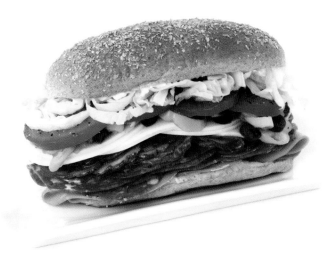

Plentiful Italian Sub

Serves 4

4 Oroweat 100% Whole Wheat Hot Dog Buns
4 Tbsp. Dijon mustard
4 Tbsp. mayonnaise
8 slices mortadella
8 slices capicola
12 slices hard salami
8 slices provolone
2 Tbsp. sliced pepperoncinis
¼ cup sliced black olives
8 thin slices of tomato
2 cups shredded iceberg lettuce
4 tsp. red-wine vinegar
1 tsp. Lawry's Seasoned Pepper or
    Lemon Pepper

1. Separate the buns and spread mustard and mayonnaise on each half. Build sandwiches by layering the bottom bun with mortadella, capicola, salami, provolone, pepperoncinis, sliced olives, tomatoes, and shredded lettuce. Drizzle with vinegar and sprinkle with seasoning; add the top bun and serve.

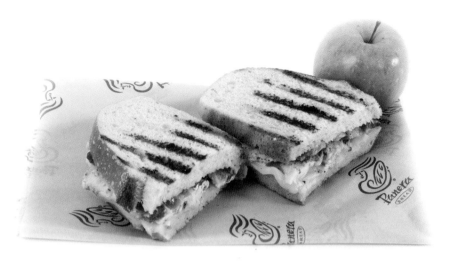

BELLY BAD

S/C Value = 29/6

BELLY GOOD

S/C Value = 3/2

Panera Bread Chicken Bacon Dijon Panini

A simple lunch of a sandwich and fruit will sabotage more than 2 days on the Belly Fat Cure if you're not smart. One apple has 15 grams of sugar alone!

Chicken Bacon Dijon Panini Do-Over:

A panini is a type of sandwich that's grilled until the ingredients are warmed. Serve it with blackberries; this antioxidant-rich fruit has less than 2 grams of sugar.

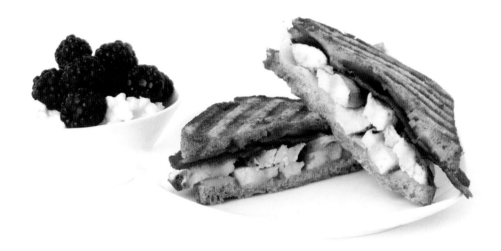

Crispy Chicken Panini

Serves 4

Sandwich:

1 Tbsp. extra-virgin olive oil

½ cup thinly sliced onion

3 cloves garlic, finely chopped

2 large chicken breasts, cooked and sliced

8 strips of turkey bacon, cooked and cut in half

8 slices Food for Life Ezekiel 4:9 Sprouted 100% Whole Grain Bread

4 Tbsp. mayonnaise

8 slices provolone

4 Tbsp. butter, softened

Other sides:

1 cup cottage cheese

1 cup blackberries

1. In a medium skillet, heat oil over medium heat. Add the onions and garlic and sauté until caramelized (about 15–20 minutes). Remove from heat and set aside.

2. Preheat a grill pan or heavy bottom skillet over medium heat (or use a panini press, following the manufacturer's instructions). Lay out 2 slices of bread per sandwich and spread each with mayonnaise. Build sandwiches by layering the bottom slice of bread with 2 slices of cheese, chicken, caramelized onions, bacon, and the top slice of bread. Lightly butter the outsides of the sandwich and place in the grill pan. Top the sandwich with a second skillet that's holding a couple of cans from your pantry to press the sandwiches down. Press the sandwiches until crisp and golden, about 2–3 minutes per side.

3. Cut the sandwiches on the diagonal and serve hot with a side of cottage cheese and blackberries.

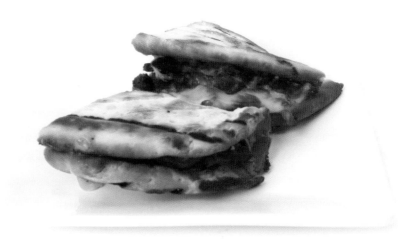

BELLY BAD

S/C Value = 14/5

Uno Chicago Grill
Southwest Steak Panini

The spread on this panini, made from cilantro and sun-dried tomato, kicks up the sugar—and the onions push it overboard. Opt for the traditional buffalo wings at Uno instead: they have just 2 grams of sugar and 6 carbs per serving.

BELLY GOOD

S/C Value = 1/2

Steak Panini
Do-Over:

Grill your own peppers: Cut them in half and place them on the grill for 8–10 minutes. Peel off the charred skin and slice. Three pepper rings add just 1 gram of sugar.

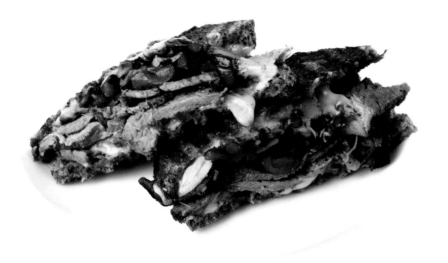

Rustic Steak & Cheese Panini

Serves 4

1 Tbsp. extra-virgin olive oil
3 cloves garlic, finely chopped
1 cup sliced portobello mushrooms
⅓ cup roasted red peppers, cut into strips
8 slices Food for Life Ezekiel 4:9 Sprouted
    100% Whole Grain Bread
4 Tbsp. mayonnaise
8 slices cheddar or Monterey Jack cheese
2 (8-oz.) New York strip steaks, cooked to
    desired doneness and sliced
4 Tbsp. butter

1. Heat the oil in a medium skillet over medium heat. Add the garlic, mushrooms, and red peppers and sauté for 3–5 minutes or until fragrant and the mushrooms are cooked. Set aside.

2. Preheat a grill pan or heavy bottom skillet over medium heat (or use a panini press, following the manufacturer's instructions). Lay out 2 slices of bread per sandwich and spread each with mayonnaise. Build sandwiches by layering the bottom slice of bread with a slice of cheese, sliced steak, sautéed vegetables, another slice of cheese, and the top slice of bread. Lightly butter the outsides of the sandwich and place in the grill pan. Top the sandwich with a second skillet that's holding a couple of cans from your pantry to press the sandwiches down. Press the sandwiches until crisp and golden, about 2–3 minutes per side.

3. Cut sandwiches on the diagonal and serve.

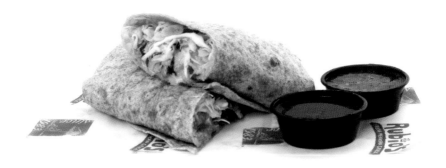

BELLY BAD

S/C Value = 18/5

Rubio's Tropical Wrapsalada

Cranberries and
a mandarin dressing
give this wrap 18
grams of sugar—
3 more than I recommend
per day if you want to look
your best and lose belly fat.

BELLY GOOD

S/C Value = 2/2

Tropical Wrap Do-Over:

One Tumaro's Garden
Spinach & Vegetables
Tortilla has just 23 grams of
carbs and 2 grams of sugar,
and it contains no trans fats.
(You can find them on
Amazon.com.)

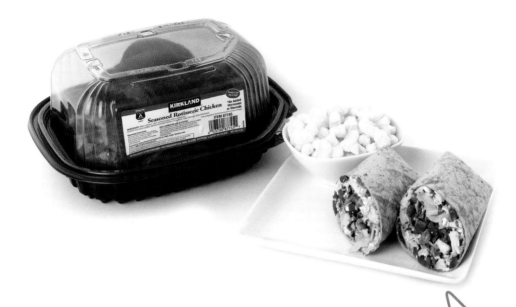

Chicken Caesar Salad Wrap

Serves 4

Wrap:
8 Tbsp. mayonnaise
2 cloves garlic, minced
1 tsp. anchovy paste
1 tsp. Worcestershire sauce
1 Tbsp. fresh lemon juice
1 tsp. Dijon mustard
¼ cup extra-virgin olive oil
4 cups shredded romaine lettuce
2 cups rotisserie chicken—white meat, no skin
    —shredded (I used the Kirkland brand)
½ cup grated Parmesan cheese
1 cup diced tomatoes
4 (8") Tumaro's Garden Spinach & Vegetables
    Tortillas

Other sides:
2 oz. Pirate's Booty Aged White Cheddar Snack

1. Place the first 7 ingredients in a blender; mix thoroughly to create a dressing. Place the shredded lettuce in a large mixing bowl and toss with the dressing, adding a little at a time so as not to overdress. Then add the chicken, cheese, diced tomatoes, and re-toss; add more dressing if needed. Divide between wraps and roll up.

2. Serve each wrap with equal amounts of Pirate's Booty.

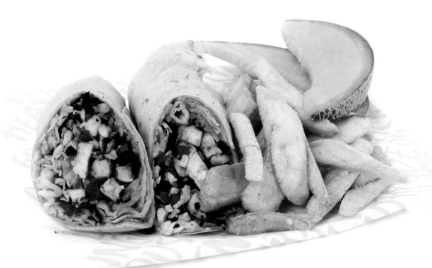

BELLY BAD

S/C Value = 33/6

Red Robin Whiskey River BBQ Chicken Wrap

According to the menu, this wrap is "smothered" in barbecue sauce, so it's easy to see how it has more than 2 days' worth of sugar on the Belly Fat Cure.

BELLY GOOD

S/C Value = 4/2

BBQ Chicken Wrap Do-Over:

You can smother all you want if you make a smarter choice. Try Scott's Barbecue Sauce—it's a 0/0.

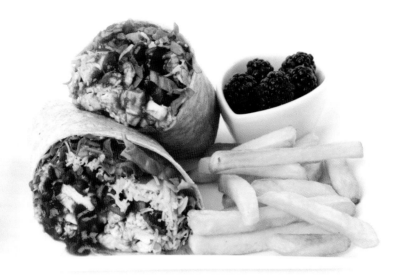

Super Tangy Chicken Wrap

Serves 4

Wrap:
4 La Tortilla Factory Smart & Delicious Multi
    Grain SoftWraps
2 cups chopped red-leaf lettuce
½ cup chopped red onion
1 cup shredded cheddar cheese
1 cup canned Progresso Black Beans, drained
4 chicken breasts, cooked and shredded
½ cup Scott's Barbecue Sauce

Other sides:
3 oz. Cascadian Farm Straight Cut French Fries,
    cooked
1 cup blackberries

1. Warm up the wraps over a gas flame or in a
pan until pliable. Layer the lettuce, onion, cheese,
beans, and chicken on one half of the tortilla. Drizzle
with barbecue sauce and roll up.

2. Serve each wrap with equal amounts of French
fries and blackberries.

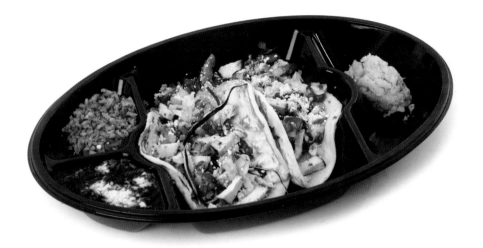

BELLY BAD

S/C Value = 14/8

Chevys Grilled Chicken Tacos

This chicken-taco plate has more carbs than you should have in an entire day. Don't worry—you can still enjoy a complete taco plate if you use the right ingredients.

BELLY GOOD

S/C Value = 4/2

Grilled Chicken Tacos Do-Over:

These tacos are stuffed with goodness and served with all of the sides, and it still earns just a 4/2. Here I also use Progresso Black Beans and Uncle Ben's rice.

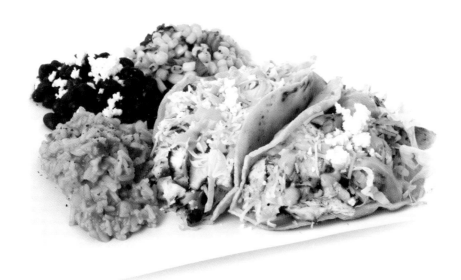

Chipotle Chicken Tacos

Serves 4

Tacos:
¼ cup extra-virgin olive oil
1 tsp. cumin
Juice of 1 lime, plus zest
1 jalapeño, stemmed, seeded, and diced
4 chicken breasts
8 (6") Mission Yellow Corn Tortillas
½ cup finely shredded cabbage
1 cup shredded Mexican blend cheese
¼ cup cilantro, chopped

Chipotle crema:
½ cup mayonnaise
¼ cup sour cream
½ Tbsp. minced garlic
½ lime, juiced
1 Tbsp. chipotle peppers in adobo sauce, minced

Other sides:
½ cup corn
2 Tbsp. butter
½ cup canned Progresso Black Beans, drained
½ cup cooked Uncle Ben's Country Inn Mexican
   Fiesta Rice

1. For the tacos: Mix the first 4 ingredients in a large Ziploc bag; add chicken breasts to marinate for at least 20 minutes. Preheat grill to medium-high heat. Remove the chicken from the marinade and discard the marinade. Pat the chicken dry with a paper towel; grill 5–7 minutes per side or until done. Remove and dice and place in a bowl.

2. For chipotle crema: Combine all listed ingredients and mix thoroughly.

3. Warm the tortillas over a gas flame or in a pan; fill with chicken, cabbage, and cheese. Top with chipotle crema and garnish with cilantro.

4. Season and heat the corn, beans, and rice; serve with the tacos.

CARB SWAP

TACOS

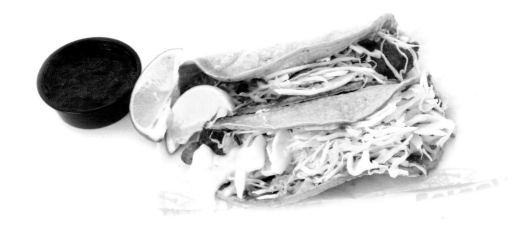

BELLY BAD

S/C Value = 8/3

Rubio's Fish Tacos Especial

Three chicken Street Tacos at Rubio's have a 3/2 S/C Value—choose them instead if you want to live the Belly Fat Cure lifestyle and look your best.

BELLY GOOD

S/C Value = 5/2

Fish Tacos Do-Over:

The Mexican version of a fish sandwich, grilled tacos are a fast-food staple of the Southwest. I like to use cod, a light white fish that cooks quickly.

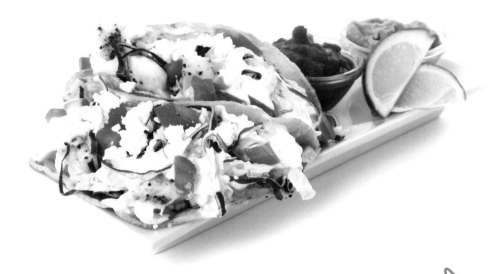

Seaside Tacos

Serves 4

Salsa crema:
½ cup mayonnaise
½ cup sour cream
½ Tbsp. minced garlic
½ lime, juiced

Guacamole:
1 avocado, mashed
½ lime, juiced
½ tsp. garlic powder

Tacos:
¼ cup chopped onions
¼ cup finely chopped cilantro
½ cup chopped tomato
8 oz. Pacific cod
8 (6") Mission Yellow or White Corn Tortillas
1 cup shredded red cabbage
½ cup crumbled cotija cheese

Other sides:
8 Tbsp. La Victoria Salsa Suprema
1 lime, cut into 8 wedges

1. For the salsa crema: Combine all listed ingredients and mix thoroughly.

2. For the guacamole: Mash the avocado with lime juice and garlic powder in a separate bowl.

3. For the tacos: Preheat grill to medium heat. Combine the onions, cilantro, and tomato in a bowl; mix and set aside. Season the cod as desired; grill for 3–4 minutes on each side or until the fish flakes easily with a fork; set aside. **Note:** When grilling fish, make sure that the grate is very clean and well oiled.

4. Warm the tortillas over a gas flame or in a pan; fill with cabbage, cilantro mix, and fish. Top with 1 Tbsp. salsa crema and cotija cheese.

5. Serve tacos with 2 lime wedges and sides of guacamole and salsa.

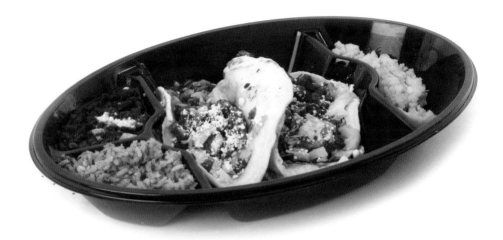

BELLY BAD

S/C Value = 14/8

Chevys Grilled Steak Tacos

The side of beans alone served with this dish has nearly 1,000 milligrams of sodium. Skip the tacos, too, because of their 14 grams of belly fat–promoting sugar.

BELLY GOOD

S/C Value = 4/2

Grilled Steak Tacos Do-Over:

Carne asada means "roasted meat" in Spanish. Use a thin steak that's easy to cut into strips, like flank or skirt steak.

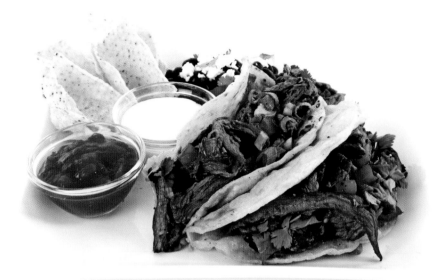

Jorge's Carne Asada Tacos

Serves 4

Tacos:
2 lbs. flank steak
1 Tbsp. McCormick Grill Mates Mesquite
    Seasoning
8 (6") Mission Yellow or White Corn Tortillas
½ cup chopped green onions
½ cup chopped tomato
½ cup finely chopped cilantro

Other sides:
½ cup canned Progresso Black Beans, drained
¼ cup La Victoria Salsa Suprema
¼ cup sour cream
24 Mission Restaurant Style Tortilla Triangles

1. For the tacos: Preheat grill to medium-high heat. Season the steak with grill seasoning. When the grill is hot, cook the steak for 3–5 minutes per side. Remove from the grill and let rest for 5 minutes; then slice across the grain of the meat.

2. Warm each tortilla over a gas flame or in a pan; fill with steak, tomato, and green onion. Garnish with cilantro.

3. Warm the beans and serve with the tacos, along with some chips and sides of sour cream and salsa.

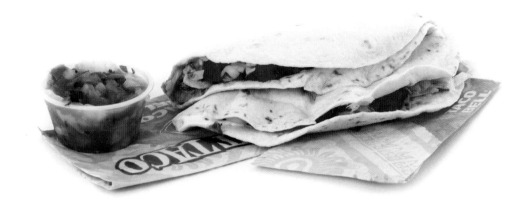

BELLY BAD

S/C Value = 8/3

Taco Bell
Soft Taco Supreme

Taco Bell has several
options that have a
5/2 or less S/C Value,
but the Taco Supreme
isn't one of them. Check
out page 313 for Belly Fat
Cure–approved items.

BELLY GOOD

S/C Value = 5/2

Taco Supreme
Do-Over:

The ground-beef taco
is more Tex-Mex than
Mexican and gained
popularity in the border
regions. Top with
fresh jalapeño slices
if you want more heat.

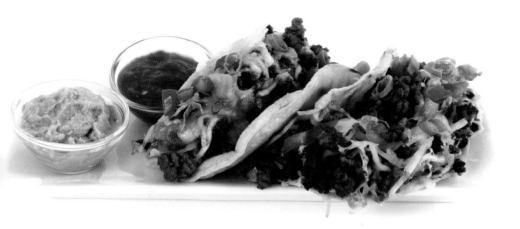

Great Ground-Beef Tacos

Serves 4

Tacos:
1 Tbsp. chili powder
1 tsp. cumin seed
1 tsp. cayenne pepper
1 Tbsp. extra-virgin olive oil
1 small jalapeño, diced
3 cloves garlic, finely chopped
¼ cup chopped onions
1 lb. lean ground beef
1 cup shredded Mexican cheese blend
1 cup shredded iceberg lettuce
½ cup chopped green onions
½ cup diced tomato
¼ cup finely chopped cilantro
8 (6") Mission Yellow Corn Tortillas

Other sides:
8 Tbsp. La Victoria Salsa Suprema
4 Tbsp. sour cream
8 Tbsp. Wholly Guacamole

1. For the tacos: In a large skillet, toast spices over medium-high heat for 1 minute or until fragrant. Add oil to the pan. Sauté the jalapeño, garlic, and onions for 1 minute; crumble in the meat. Stirring frequently, cook until the meat is brown; drain and set aside.

2. Warm each tortilla over a gas flame or in a pan; fill with meat, cheese, lettuce, green onions, and tomatoes. Garnish with chopped cilantro.

3. Serve with sides of salsa and guacamole.

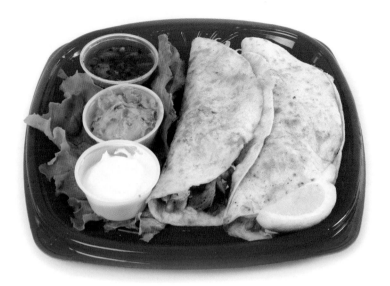

BELLY BAD

S/C Value = 12/4

Ruby's Diner Shrimp Tacos

Eating more than 5 grams of sugar at one meal programs your body to store belly fat; plus, too much sugar freezes your white blood cells' ability to fend off attackers.

BELLY GOOD

S/C Value = 5/2

Shrimp Tacos Do-Over:

We used the 6" Mission Yellow Corn Tortillas so that you can have 3 delicious shrimp tacos. Visit the food list in Chapter 6 for more recommended tortillas.

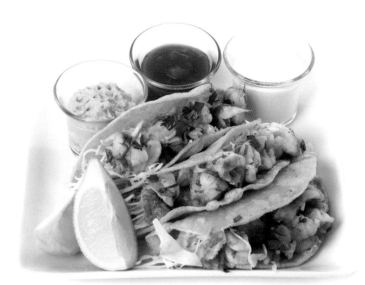

Simple Shrimp Tacos

Serves 4

Tacos:
1 lb. medium frozen, uncooked shrimp; thawed and peeled
Juice of ½ lime
3 Tbsp. butter
12 (6") Mission Yellow Corn Tortillas
1 cup finely shredded cabbage
¼ cup chopped cilantro
Tabasco Pepper Sauce, to taste

Other sides:
8 lemon wedges
8 Tbsp. La Victoria Salsa Suprema
4 Tbsp. sour cream
4 Tbsp. Wholly Guacamole

1. In a large bowl, toss the shrimp with lime juice and season to taste. Melt the butter in a large skillet over medium-high heat; add the shrimp and sauté for about 3–4 minutes or until opaque.

2. Warm the tortillas over a gas flame or in a pan; fill with shrimp and cabbage. Garnish with cilantro.

3. Serve the tacos with lemon wedges and sides of salsa, sour cream, and guacamole.

CARB SWAP

TACOS

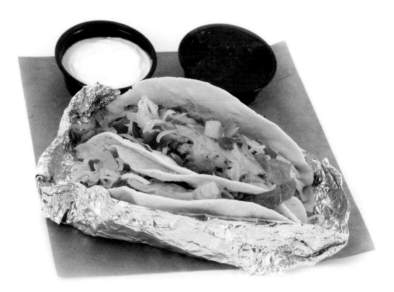

BELLY BAD

S/C Value = 5/3

BELLY GOOD

S/C Value = 4/2

Chipotle Braised Carnitas Soft Tacos

This meal from the Chipotle chain just nudges over with a 5/3. Try their chicken tacos with only cheese and lettuce for a 1/2 instead.

Carnitas Tacos Do-Over:

Carnitas is slow-cooked pork that is typically fried. The frying is skipped here, but the flavor isn't— particularly when the tacos are topped with cilantro, a type of Mexican parsley.

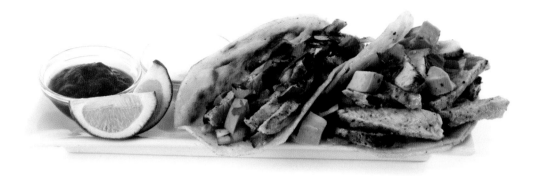

Zesty Carnitas Tacos

Serves 4

Tacos:
1½ lbs. pork shoulder
Salt and pepper to taste
Water or chicken broth, as needed
1 garlic clove, chopped
1 Tbsp. bay leaf
¼ cup chopped cilantro
¼ cup chopped red onions
1 cup lettuce, shredded
1 avocado, diced
8 (6") Mission Yellow Corn Tortillas

Other sides:
8 lemon wedges
8 Tbsp. sour cream
8 Tbsp. La Victoria Salsa Suprema

1. Season the pork with salt and pepper and cut into a few pieces; place in a deep pot. Fill with broth or water 1" above the pork; add the bay leaf and garlic. Bring to a boil, then reduce heat to a simmer and cover. Continue simmering for 1½–2½ hours or until the pork falls apart easily; check the level of the liquid periodically and add more if necessary. When the pork is done, let it cool enough to handle and shred.

2. Warm the tortillas over a gas flame or in a pan; fill with shredded pork, lettuce, onion, cilantro, and avocado.

3. Serve tacos with lime wedges and sides of sour cream and salsa.

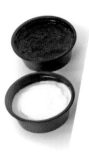
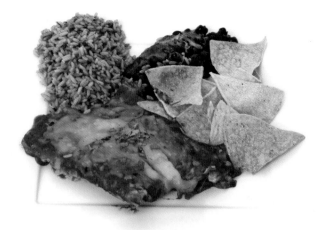

BELLY BAD

S/C Value = 10/6

La Salsa Cheese Enchilada Platter

This meal might fill you up, but it will also fill out your waistline. Keep in mind that 10 grams of sugar is ⅔ of your day on the Belly Fat Cure—skip it.

BELLY GOOD

S/C Value = 3/2

Enchilada Platter Do-Over:

This incredible dish has an S/C Value of just 3/2. Eat smarter meals like this every day and you will lose belly fat and look your best.

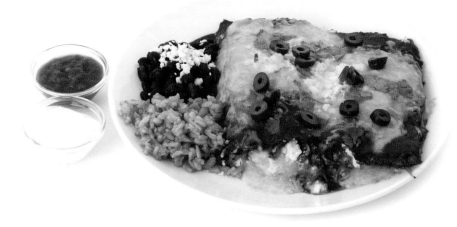

Cheesy Enchiladas

Serves 4

Enchiladas:

½ (10 oz.) can La Victoria Red Enchilada Sauce, divided use

8 Tbsp. cream cheese, softened or whipped

8 (6") Mission Yellow or White Corn Tortillas

1 cup baby spinach leaves

1 cup crumbled cotija or feta cheese, divided use

1 cup grated cheese of your choice, divided (reserve half to sprinkle on enchiladas)

½ cup chopped green onions

4 Tbsp. sliced black olives, for serving

½ cup chopped cilantro, for serving

Other sides:

1 cup canned Progresso Black Beans, drained

2 Tbsp. chopped cilantro

1 tsp. Mrs. Dash Extra Spicy Seasoning Blend

½ cup Uncle Ben's Country Inn Mexican Fiesta Rice, cooked

4 Tbsp. sour cream

4 Tbsp. La Victoria Salsa Suprema

1. Preheat oven to 425° F. Pour half of the enchilada sauce into a pie plate or baking dish. Warm the tortillas over a gas flame or in a pan, and dip in the enchilada sauce. Spread cream cheese on each tortilla; divide and add the spinach, ¾ cup of the cotija cheese, half of the grated cheese, and the green onions down the center. Roll up the tortillas and place in a baking dish, seam-side down. Pour the remainder of the enchilada sauce over the top, and sprinkle the reserved shredded cheese evenly over that.

2. Cover with foil and bake for 20 minutes or until the cheese is melted. Remove from the oven, and top with cilantro and olives.

3. Heat the beans with cilantro and seasoning, and cook the rice.

4. Garnish the enchiladas and black beans with the remaining cotija cheese. Serve with cooked rice and sides of sour cream and salsa.

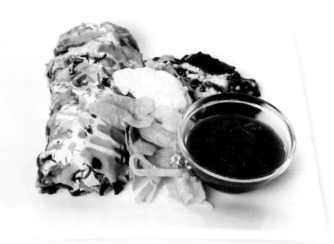

BELLY BAD

S/C Value = 15/4

Mimi's Café Smokey Chicken Enchiladas

This chain has a few meals on our Belly Bad list—the worst of which is their banana chocolate chip pancakes. While these enchiladas aren't that bad, they do have too much sugar for a single meal.

BELLY GOOD

S/C Value = 3/2

Smokey Chicken Enchiladas Do-Over:

The green enchilada sauce from La Victoria adds no sugar to this dish. Top with cotija cheese, a Mexican cheese similar to feta that adds delicious flavor.

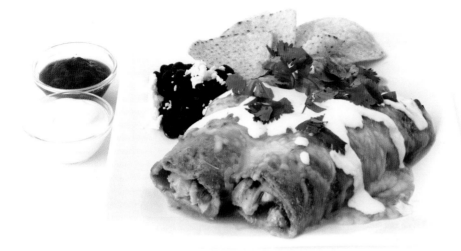

Superb Chicken Enchiladas

Serves 4

Enchiladas:
2 large chicken breasts
1 tsp. salt
8 (6") Mission Yellow or White Corn Tortillas
8 Tbsp. cream cheese, softened or whipped
½ (10 oz.) can La Victoria Green Enchilada Sauce
1 cup crumbled cotija cheese, divided use
1 cup grated cheese of your choice, divided
¼ cup sour cream, for serving
½ cup chopped green onions, for serving

Other sides:
½ cup canned Progresso Black Beans, drained
2 Tbsp. chopped cilantro
1 Tbsp. Mrs. Dash Extra Spicy Seasoning Blend
16 Mission Restaurant Style Tortilla Triangles
¼ cup sour cream
¼ cup La Victoria Salsa Suprema

1. Preheat oven to 425° F. Add salt and chicken to a pot of water; bring to a boil. Reduce heat to simmer for 15 minutes. Remove chicken; shred once it's cool enough to handle. Pour half of the enchilada sauce into a pie plate or baking dish. Warm the tortillas over a gas flame or in a pan, then dip in the enchilada sauce. Spread cream cheese on each tortilla, then divide and add the shredded chicken, ¾ cup of the cotija cheese, half of the grated cheese, and the green onions down the center. Roll up the tortillas and place in a baking dish, seam-side down. Pour the remainder of the enchilada sauce over the top, and sprinkle with the reserved shredded cheese.

2. Cover with foil and bake for 20 minutes or until the cheese is melted. Remove from the oven, and top with sour cream and cilantro.

3. Heat the beans with cilantro and seasoning.

4. Garnish the enchiladas and black beans with the remaining cotija cheese. Serve with some chips and sides of sour cream and salsa.

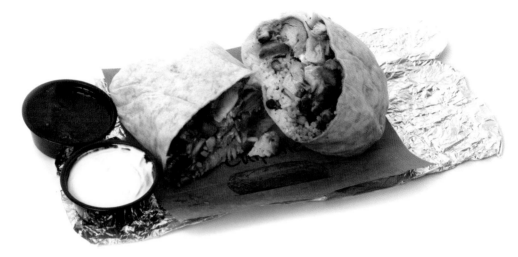

BELLY BAD

S/C Value = 7/4

Chipotle Grilled Chicken Burrito

With 80 grams of carbs, this gets a 4 on the S/C Value. It would take up more than half of your carbs *and* about half of your sugars in one sitting.

BELLY GOOD

S/C Value = 3/2

Chicken Burrito Do-Over:

This recipe calls for baking your own chicken, but you can also use a store-bought rotisserie chicken instead to cut back on cooking time.

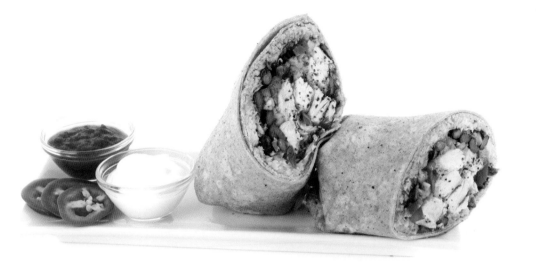

Seasoned Chicken Burrito

Serves 4

Burrito:
4 large chicken breasts
Salt and pepper, to taste
½ cup canned Progresso Black Beans, drained
4 La Tortilla Factory Organic Wheat Tortillas, Low Fat, Carb Cutting
1 cup Uncle Ben's Country Inn Mexican Fiesta Rice, cooked
1 cup shredded Mexican cheese blend
1 cup shredded iceberg lettuce
½ cup chopped onions
¼ cup chopped cilantro
1 jalapeño, seeded and finely chopped
½ cup chopped tomatoes
1 avocado, diced

Other sides:
½ cup La Victoria Salsa Suprema
4 Tbsp. sour cream

1. Preheat oven to 400° F. Season the chicken with salt and pepper and place in the oven for 20–25 minutes or until done. Remove chicken and slice.

2. Heat the beans in a small pan. Warm the tortillas over a gas flame or in a pan. Divide the cooked rice and add it down the center of each tortilla; top with the sliced chicken, cheese, lettuce, beans, onion, cilantro, jalapeño, tomato, and avocado. Fold up the bottom part of the tortilla, then roll each side over. Serve each with a side of salsa and sour cream.

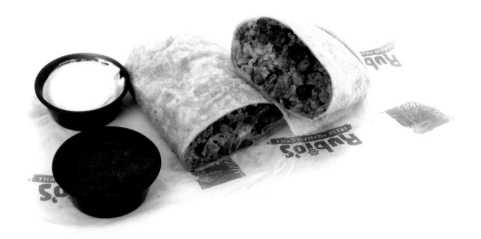

BELLY BAD

S/C Value = 8/7

Rubio's Big Burrito Especial

This burrito has more carbs than steak, which is why it has nearly 100 carbohydrate grams (not counting chips). A creamy chipotle sauce adds 8 grams of sugar, too.

BELLY GOOD

S/C Value = 3/2

Big Burrito Especial Do-Over:

This is how to properly make a burrito: Add filling to a tortilla and fold the bottom up. Flip the right side over and then wrap the left side over that. Finish by closing the top piece like a lid.

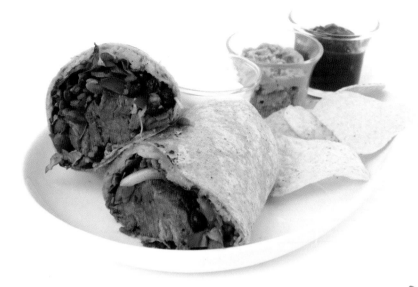

Round 'em Up Steak Burrito

Serves 4

Burrito:

2 Tbsp. extra-virgin olive oil
2 (8-oz.) New York steaks
2 cloves garlic, finely chopped
¼ cup chopped onion
¼ cup chopped cilantro
1 jalapeño, seeded and finely chopped
1 tsp. ground cumin
½ cup canned Progresso Black Beans, drained
4 La Tortilla Factory Organic Wheat Tortillas, Low Fat, Carb Cutting
1 cup Uncle Ben's Country Inn Mexican Fiesta Rice, cooked
1 cup shredded Mexican blend cheese
½ cup shredded green-leaf lettuce
½ cup chopped tomatoes

Other sides:

3 Tbsp. La Victoria Salsa Suprema
4 Tbsp. Wholly Guacamole
4 Tbsp. sour cream
20 Mission Restaurant Style Tortilla Triangles

1. Slice the steaks into ½" strips. Heat the oil in a large skillet over medium-high heat. When the oil is hot, add the steak and sauté for 1 minute. Add the next 5 ingredients and continue to sauté until the meat is cooked to your liking.

2. Heat the beans in a small pan. Warm the tortillas over a gas flame or in a pan. Divide the cooked rice and add it down the center of each tortilla; top with the steak mixture, cheese, lettuce, beans, and tomato. Fold up the bottom part of the tortilla, then roll each side over. Serve with sides of salsa, guacamole, sour cream, and chips.

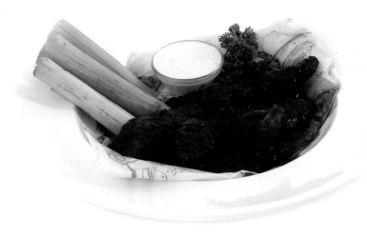

BELLY BAD

S/C Value = 17/4

Denny's Chicken Strips

Even though this dish is just an appetizer, it has more than a day's worth of sugar on the Belly Fat Cure and 4 servings of carbs.

BELLY GOOD

S/C Value = 2/1

Chicken Strips Do-Over:

This easy meal is perfect for game night or slumber parties—just be sure to pass out plenty of napkins. You get 3 pieces of chicken per serving and a great dip, all for a 2/1.

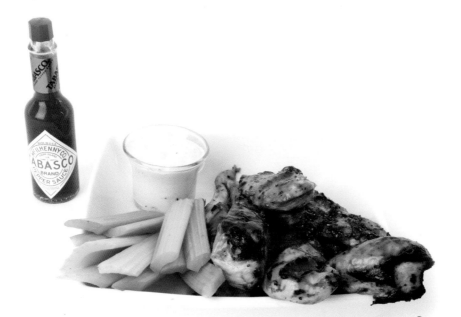

Owen's Finger-Lickin' Chicken Strips   Serves 4

Chicken strips:
4 large chicken breasts
Salt and pepper, to taste
½ cup Scott's Barbecue Sauce
Tabasco Pepper Sauce, to taste
2 tsp. chili powder
¼ tsp. ground cayenne pepper

Blue-cheese dip:
½ cup mayonnaise
¼ cup extra-virgin olive oil
2 Tbsp. red-wine vinegar
1 tsp. Dijon mustard
½ cup blue-cheese crumbles
1 tsp. finely chopped shallots

Other sides:
4 celery sticks, cut into 4" pieces
Tabasco Pepper Sauce, for serving

1. For the chicken: Preheat oven to 400° F. Layer a baking sheet with aluminum foil. Cut each chicken breast lengthwise into 3 even pieces, for a total of 12 pieces. Season as desired and put in the oven for 15–20 minutes or until done. Stir together the barbecue sauce, Tabasco, chili powder, and cayenne pepper. When the chicken is ready, brush barbecue mixture on both sides until coated, and place it back in the oven for 2 more minutes.

2. For the blue-cheese dip: Mix the listed ingredients in a food processor until smooth.

3. Serve the chicken strips with a side of blue-cheese dip and celery—and be sure to leave the bottle of Tabasco on the table!

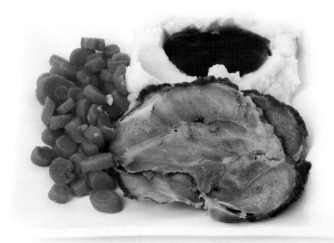

BELLY BAD

S/C Value = 10/3

BELLY GOOD

S/C Value = 3/2

Hometown Buffet Holiday Meal

Swap the carrots with green beans and you knock out 6 grams of sugar. See page 306 for the best and worst veggies on the Belly Fat Cure.

Holiday Meal Do-Over:

Make candied carrots with stevia instead of sugar; the herbal sweetener lets you enjoy this holiday treat without the consequence of belly fat.

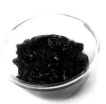

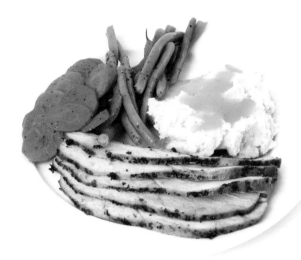

The Best Holiday Dinner

Serves 4

Turkey:
2 lbs. boneless, skinless turkey breast; 4 Tbsp. butter; 1½ tsp. Tabasco Pepper Sauce; 2 Tbsp. fresh rosemary, finely chopped; 2 tsp. thyme, finely chopped; 2 Tbsp. Mrs. Dash Lemon Pepper Seasoning Blend; 1 Tbsp. paprika

Carrots:
4 Tbsp. butter; 2 packets stevia; 1 cup sliced carrots; ¼ cup chicken broth

Cranberry sauce:
1 cup fresh cranberries, rinsed; 2 packets stevia (or more, to taste); ½ cup water; 1 tsp. finely chopped orange zest; 1 tsp. cinnamon; 1 tsp. nutmeg

Green beans:
1 cup green beans; 2 Tbsp. butter

Other sides:
1 cup Heinz Rich Mushroom HomeStyle Gravy; 1 cup prepared Ore-Ida Steam n' Mash Garlic Seasoned Potatoes; Mrs. Dash Lemon Pepper Seasoning Blend, to taste, for serving

1. For the turkey: Preheat oven to 350° F. Melt the butter and Tabasco in a pot. Place the turkey in a pan, skin-side up. Loosen the skin and place the rosemary and thyme under the skin as well as under the breast. Baste the turkey with the butter and Tabasco; season with lemon pepper and paprika, and add other seasonings as desired. Cook for approximately 60–70 minutes or until the internal temperature reads 160° F. Remove the turkey from the oven, tent with foil, and let rest for 10 minutes.

2. For the carrots: In a medium skillet, combine the butter and stevia over medium heat until bubbling; add the carrots and sauté until tender. Add chicken broth and cook until most of the liquid has evaporated.

3. For the cranberry sauce: Combine all of the ingredients in a small pan and bring to a boil. Reduce heat and simmer for about 30 minutes, until the water has reduced somewhat.

4. For the green beans: Boil the beans for 5 minutes in a medium saucepan; drain and sauté in butter.

5. For the potatoes: Prepare according to package directions.

6. Slice the turkey and top the potatoes with gravy. Serve with carrots, green beans, and cranberry sauce.

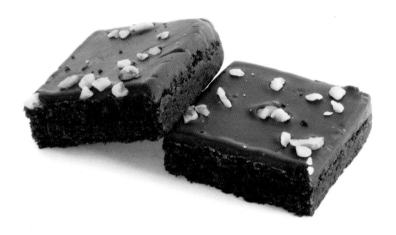

BELLY BAD

S/C Value = 21/2

BELLY GOOD

S/C Value = 0/1

Little Debbie Fudge Brownies

Eat a few of these Little Debbie brownies and there will be *nothing* little about your waistline! With 21 grams of sugar, there's more sugar in 1 brownie than I recommend you eat in an entire day.

Fudge Brownies Do-Over:

This delicious brownie has a nice light texture and indulgently rich chocolate flavor. Enjoy as a tasty special-occasion dessert, or have it as often as you like—it has no sugar!

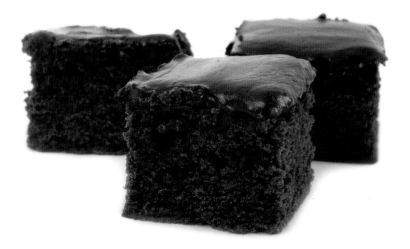

Outrageous Chocolate Brownie

Serves 16

Brownie:

¾ cup unsalted butter, softened

1½ cups Joseph's Maltitol Sweetener syrup
  (see p. 262)

1½ tsp. vanilla extract

3 eggs

¾ cup flour

½ cup cocoa

½ tsp. baking powder

½ tsp. salt

Optional Glaze:

½ cup heavy cream

2 oz. unsweetened baking chocolate

¼ cup maltitol sweetener syrup

2–5 packets Truvia, to taste

1. For the brownies: Preheat oven to 350° F. Butter an 8" square pan. In a bowl, blend softened butter with maltitol syrup and vanilla. Add eggs and beat well. Combine flour, cocoa, baking powder and salt. Add to egg mixture and stir until well blended. Pour batter into prepared pan and bake for 40–45 minutes. Cool completely.

2. For the glaze: Heat cream and chocolate over low heat and stir frequently until melted. Remove from heat and whisk in maltitol syrup until smooth. Add Truvia one packet at a time to taste.

3. Pour glaze over the brownies and let set before cutting into 2" squares.

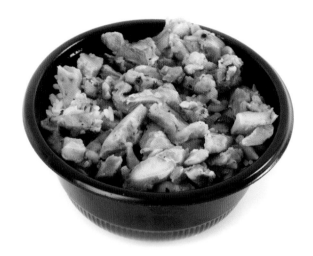

BELLY BAD

S/C Value = 8/5

Panda Express Mandarin Chicken Panda Bowl with Steamed Rice

Try the Kung Pao Chicken or Broccoli Beef instead; both have just 3 grams of sugar. And skip the white rice—it has too many carbs and no nutritional value.

BELLY GOOD

S/C Value = 4/2

Chicken with Steamed Rice Do-Over:

The more colors you can work into your diet, the better; they represent a variety of phytochemicals and antioxidants found in different fruits and vegetables.

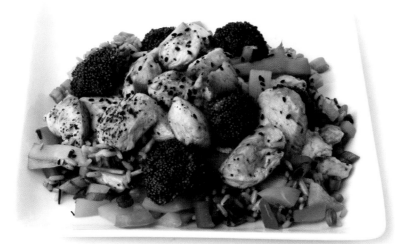

Chicken Sesame Stir-Fry

Serves 4

Teriyaki Dressing:
½ cup low-sodium soy sauce
Juice from ½ orange
2 tsp. stevia
¼ tsp. garlic powder
1/8 tsp. ground ginger
2 tsp. sesame oil

Stir-Fry:
1 Tbsp. vegetable oil
2 large chicken breasts, cut into bite-size pieces
3 cloves garlic, finely chopped
1 cup broccoli florets
½ cup canned bamboo shoots, drained
½ cup chopped red bell peppers
½ cup chopped yellow bell peppers
½ cup chopped orange bell peppers
½ cup thinly sliced green onions
1 Tbsp. black sesame seeds

Other sides:
2 cups Uncle Ben's Fast & Natural Whole Grain
   Instant Brown Rice, cooked

1. For the teriyaki dressing: Combine all of the ingredients in a small saucepan. Bring to a boil over medium-high heat, stirring constantly; continue cooking until the mixture thickens slightly. Remove and set aside.

2. For the stir-fry: Heat a large skillet over medium-high heat; add the vegetable oil. When the oil is shimmering, add the chicken and garlic, and stir-fry for 2–3 minutes. Add the broccoli and continue to stir-fry for 4–6 minutes. Add the bamboo shoots and peppers and cook for an additional 4–6 minutes. Carefully pour in the teriyaki dressing (watch for splattering); cook until the chicken is cooked through and the vegetables are done to your liking. Remove from heat and stir in the green onions and sesame seeds, reserving some of each for garnishing.

3. Serve immediately over cooked rice garnished with the reserved green onions and sesame seeds.

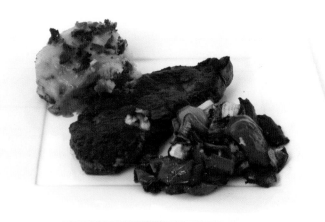

BELLY BAD

S/C Value = 20/4

Uno Chicago Grill Brewmaster's Grill NY Sirloin Steak

Sticking to 15 grams a day of sugar will help you lose belly fat fast and keep your immune system strong; that means that 20 grams in a single meal, like this one, is too much.

BELLY GOOD

S/C Value = 3/2

Sirloin Steak Do-Over:

Asparagus is an excellent source of folate, which is good for your heart and critical if you're thinking about conceiving; low levels have been linked to birth defects.

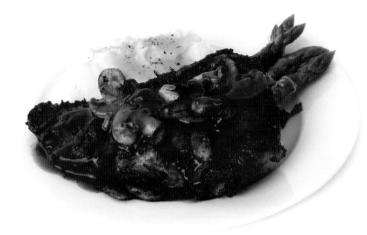

Gourmet Grilled Steak

Serves 4

Steak:
4 (8-oz.) sirloin steaks
Salt and pepper, to taste

Mushroom gravy:
2 Tbsp. butter
1 cup sliced white mushrooms
3 cloves garlic, minced
2 tsp. fresh rosemary, finely chopped
1 cup Heinz Rich Mushroom HomeStyle Gravy
2 Tbsp. red wine

Asparagus:
1 Tbsp. extra-virgin olive oil
20 medium-size asparagus spears
Salt and pepper, to taste

Other Sides:
2 cups prepared Ore-Ida Steam n' Mash
    Three Cheese Potatoes

1. For the steak: Preheat oven to 375° F. Preheat grill to medium-high heat. Season meat as desired. When the grill is hot, grill the steaks for 5 minutes on each side or to desired doneness.

2. For the mushroom gravy: In a skillet over medium-high heat, melt the butter. Add the mushrooms, garlic, and rosemary. Sauté until the mushrooms are golden and any liquid let off by the mushrooms has evaporated. Stir in the gravy and wine and simmer for 10 minutes.

3. For the asparagus: Lay the spears in a single layer on a sheet pan. Drizzle with olive oil and salt and pepper; toss to coat. Roast in the preheated oven for 8–10 minutes or until tender.

4. For the potatoes: Prepare according to package directions.

5. Serve the steaks and potatoes with mushroom gravy and asparagus on the side.

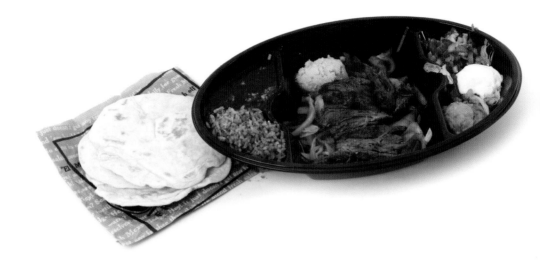

BELLY BAD

S/C Value = 19/9

Chevys Sizzling Steak Fajitas

The citrus-chili marinade makes a big contribution to the 19 grams of sugar here. I'd suggest another option at Chevys, but even their tacos have at least 5 grams of sugar.

BELLY GOOD

S/C Value = 2/2

Steak Fajitas Do-Over:

This recipe features Mission 6" Yellow Corn Tortillas, which have just 11 carb grams each; even as you enjoy rice and beans with your fajitas, this meal comes in at just a 2/2.

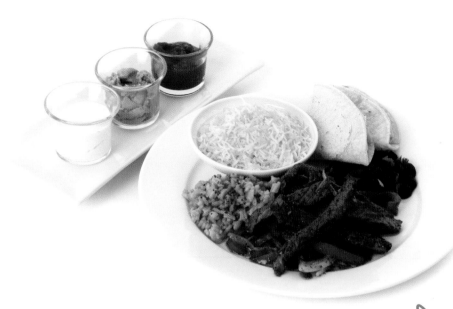

Bountiful Steak Fajitas

Serves 4

Fajitas:
16 oz. beef rib eye steak
2 Tbsp. vegetable oil
1 fresh, sliced jalapeño
½ cup sliced green bell pepper
½ cup sliced red bell pepper
½ cup julienned onion
1 tsp. cumin
1 tsp. paprika

Other sides:
8 (6") Mission Yellow Corn Tortillas
½ cup canned Progresso Black Beans, drained
½ cup Uncle Ben's Country Inn Mexican Fiesta
    Rice, cooked
4 Tbsp. sour cream
4 Tbsp. La Victoria Salsa Suprema
4 Tbsp. Wholly Guacamole

1. Slice the rib eye into thin slices. Heat a large skillet over medium-high heat; add oil. When the oil is hot, add the steak and cook for 5 minutes, stirring occasionally. Add the peppers, onions, jalapeño, and seasonings; sauté until tender.

2. Heat the beans in a small pan and warm the tortillas over a gas flame or in a pan. Serve the fajita mixture, beans, rice, and tortillas with sides of salsa, guacamole, and sour cream.

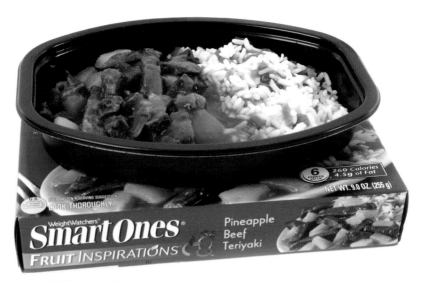

BELLY BAD

S/C Value = 15/2

BELLY GOOD

S/C Value = 5/2

Weight Watchers Smart Ones Pineapple Beef Teriyaki

Teriyaki is one of those sauces that delivers an overdose of sugar in a small amount—just 2 Tbsp. can have more than 15 grams of sugar.

Pineapple Beef Teriyaki Do-Over:

Keep the size uniform when you cut the vegetables for a stir-fry; this way, everything will cook evenly.

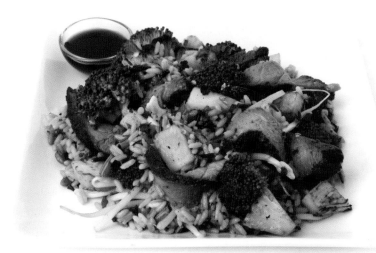

Sweet Pineapple Stir-Fry

Serves 4

Stir-Fry:
2 Tbsp. vegetable oil, divided use
4 (8-oz.) New York steaks
3 cloves garlic, finely chopped
1 Tbsp. finely chopped ginger root
½ cup chopped fresh pineapple
1 cup chopped broccoli florets
1 cup soybean sprouts
2 packets stevia
½ tsp. red pepper flakes
¼ cup low-sodium soy sauce
1 Tbsp. balsamic vinegar
2 tsp. sesame oil

Other sides:
2 cups Uncle Ben's Long Grain & Wild Rice, cooked

1. Slice the steak into thin slices. Heat a large skillet on medium-high heat; add 1 Tbsp. of the vegetable oil. When the oil is shimmering, add the steak. Stir-fry for 2 minutes, then remove with a slotted spoon and set aside. Add the remaining 1 Tbsp. of oil, along with the garlic, ginger, pineapple, and broccoli. Stir-fry for 3–5 minutes and add the remaining ingredients; cook until the broccoli reaches desired doneness. Add the steak back in the pan and toss through.

2. Serve the stir-fry immediately over rice.

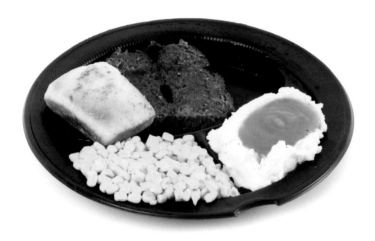

BELLY BAD

S/C Value = 28/7

Boston Market Meatloaf Individual Meal

The sweet-corn side dish has 10 grams of sugar— more than a regular serving of corn would normally have. Definitely watch for added sugars when you dine out.

BELLY GOOD

S/C Value = 3/2

Meatloaf Meal Do-Over:

Make this dish on a weekend and enjoy leftovers for lunch— or throw it in the oven as soon as you get home, and rest while your oven does the work.

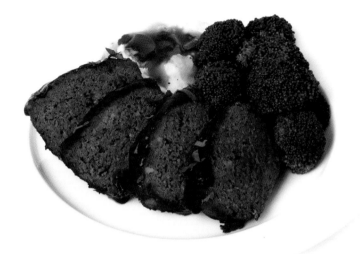

Home-Style Meatloaf

Serves 4

Meatloaf:
2 Tbsp. butter
½ cup grated carrots
½ cup chopped celery
½ cup diced onion
1 garlic clove, finely chopped
2 lbs. lean ground beef
2 large eggs
1 tsp. salt
1 tsp. pepper
1 tsp. dried oregano
2 Tbsp. Dijon mustard
½ cup Scott's Barbecue Sauce

Broccoli:
2 cups broccoli florets
2 Tbsp. butter

Other sides:
2 cups prepared Ore-Ida Steam n' Mash
   Russet Potatoes
1 cup Heinz Rich Mushroom HomeStyle Gravy

1. For the meatloaf: Preheat oven to 350° F. In a saucepan, melt the butter over medium heat and add the carrots, celery, onion, and garlic. Sauté until vegetables are done; let cool. Once cooled, add the vegetables to a large bowl along with the next 6 ingredients; mix thoroughly by hand. Press into a well-oiled loaf pan and spread barbecue sauce over the top. Bake for 1 hour or until the internal temperature reaches 150° F. Remove and let rest for 10 minutes.

2. For the broccoli: Steam the florets for 6–7 minutes; toss with butter and season as desired.

3. For the potatoes: Prepare according to package directions. Heat the gravy in a small saucepan.

4. Slice the meatloaf and serve, along with the steamed broccoli and mashed potatoes and gravy.

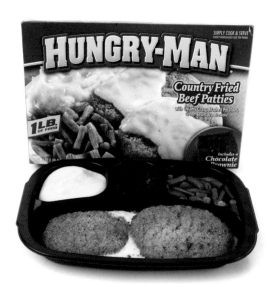

BELLY BAD

S/C Value = 24/4

BELLY GOOD

S/C Value = 2/2

Hungry-Man Country Fried Beef Patties

The 24 grams in this dish make up almost 2 days' worth of sugar on the Belly Fat Cure. Remember, more than 15 grams a day will promote belly fat and weaken your immune system.

Country Fried Beef Patties Do-Over:

I've made this dish with smarter ingredients so that the entire meal has an S/C Value of just 2/2— and that's including dessert.

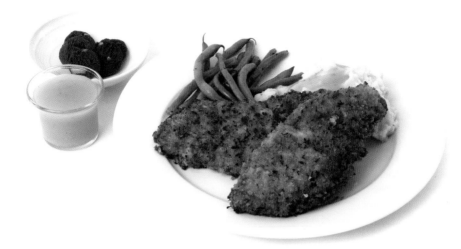

Fantastic Fried Steak

Serves 4

Steak:
3 eggs, beaten
¼ cup Arrowhead Mills Organic Soy Flour
½ cup panko (Japanese bread crumbs)
¼ Tbsp. Mrs. Dash Italian Medley Seasoning
    Blend
8 (4-oz.) pieces of cube steak
2 Tbsp. extra-virgin olive oil

Green beans:
1 cup green beans
1 Tbsp. butter

Other sides:
2 cups prepared Ore-Ida Steam n' Mash Garlic
    Seasoned Potatoes
1 cup Heinz Rich Mushroom HomeStyle Gravy
20 Joseph's Sugar-Free Bite Size Pecan Walnut
    Brownies

1. For the steak: Place the eggs, flour, and panko into three separate shallow bowls. Stir the Mrs. Dash seasoning into the flour. Dredge each piece of steak in the flour; dip into the beaten eggs and dredge in the panko. Heat the olive oil in a pan over medium-high heat. Fry the steak in batches (do not overcrowd the pan) for 4 minutes per side or until golden brown, adding more oil if necessary.

2. For the green beans: Steam the beans for 3–5 minutes; toss with butter and season as desired.

3. For the potatoes: Prepare according to package directions. Heat the gravy in a small saucepan.

4. Serve the steak, green beans, and potatoes with a side of gravy. Finish with some bite-size brownies.

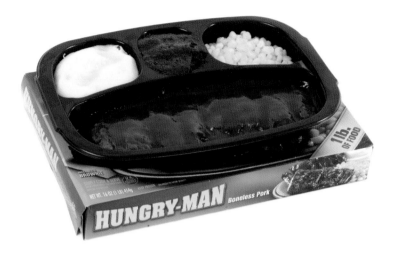

BELLY BAD

S/C Value = 76/6

Hungry-Man Boneless Pork

This meal may satisfy your appetite, like it says, but with 76 grams of sugar, it will also expand your waistline. The patties are trouble because they're soaked in high-sugar barbecue sauce.

BELLY GOOD

S/C Value = 3/2

Boneless Pork Do-Over:

Ribs are a summertime favorite; the good news is that you can enjoy them and lose belly fat, too. Use Scott's Barbecue Sauce, which has no sugar.

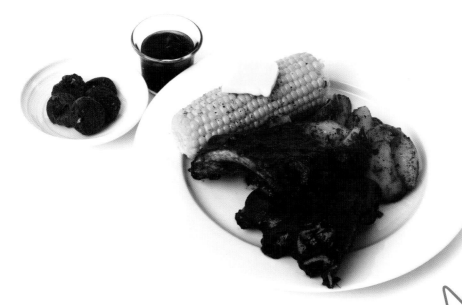

Bold Pork Spareribs

Serves 4

Spareribs:
2 lbs. pork spareribs, cut into 3-bone serving
  sections
2 Tbsp. McCormick Grill Mates Mesquite Grill
  Seasoning
1 cup Scott's Barbecue Sauce

Other sides:
4 ears corn on the cob (5½" to 6½")
1 cup Simply Potatoes Red Potato Wedges
2 Tbsp. butter
Salt and seasonings, to taste
8 Tbsp. Scott's Barbecue Sauce, for serving
16 Joseph's Sugar-Free Bite Size Pecan Walnut
  Brownies

1. For the spareribs: Place the pork in a large stock-pot and cover with water. Bring water to a boil, then reduce to a simmer for 1 hour. Remove the ribs from the water and season with mesquite seasoning. Preheat grill to medium heat. Grill the meat for 6–8 minutes total, turning every couple of minutes and brushing with barbecue sauce each time.

2. For the corn: Boil ears until tender, about 8–10 minutes. Top each ear with some butter.

3. For the potatoes: Prepare according to package directions.

4. Serve the corn, potatoes, and ribs with a side of barbecue sauce. Finish with some bite-size brownies.

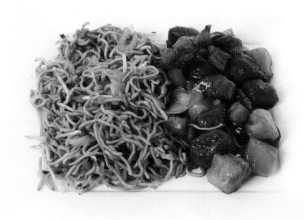

BELLY BAD

S/C Value = 41/7

Panda Express
Sweet & Sour Pork

Sweet-and-sour sauce can be made from sugar and pineapple juice or brown sugar and ketchup—these high-sugar items easily add up to almost 3 days' worth of sugar.

BELLY GOOD

S/C Value = 4/2

Sweet & Sour Pork
Do-Over:

I've re-created sweet-and-sour sauce with stevia, soy sauce, and vinegar—it's a tasty combination that gives you just a 4/2 S/C Value.

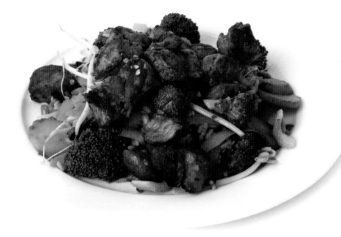

Sumptuous Pork Stir-Fry

Serves 4

Stir-fry:

1 lb. pork tenderloin, trimmed

2 Tbsp. vegetable oil

3 cloves garlic, chopped

1 cup chopped broccoli florets

½ cup sliced carrots

½ cup sliced celery

½ cup sliced water chestnuts, drained

1 cup soybean sprouts

2 packets stevia

1 tsp. red pepper flakes

¼ cup soy sauce

1 Tbsp. balsamic vinegar

2 tsp. toasted sesame oil

¼ cup green onion, chopped

Other sides:

2 cups Uncle Ben's Long Grain & Wild Rice, cooked

1. Slice the pork into bite-size pieces. Heat a large skillet over medium-high heat; add the vegetable oil and garlic. When the oil is shimmering, add the pork and stir-fry for 2–3 minutes. Add the garlic, broccoli, carrots, and celery; continue stir-frying for 4–6 minutes. Add the next 7 ingredients and cook for 5–7 minutes or until the pork is cooked through and the vegetables are tender. Remove from heat and stir in the green onions, reserving some for garnish.

2. Garnish the stir-fry with the remaining green onions and immediately serve over cooked rice.

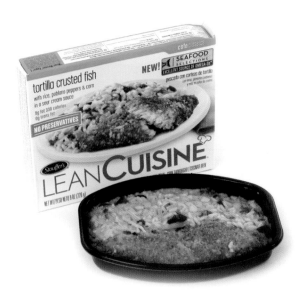

BELLY BAD

S/C Value = 7/3

BELLY GOOD

S/C Value = 1/2

Lean Cuisine
Tortilla Crusted Fish

There are more than
25 Lean Cuisine meals
I recommend, but this isn't
one of them. See the food
list in Chapter 6 for Belly Fat
Cure–approved options.

Crusted Fish
Do-Over:

Halibut is an excellent
source of omega-3 essen-
tial fatty acids, which can
lower levels of LDL (bad
cholesterol). Plus, it's an
excellent source of protein.

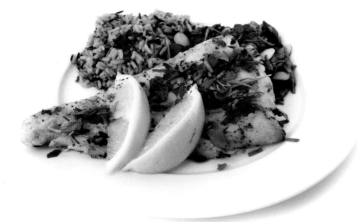

Pan-Seared Halibut

Serves 4

Fish:
4 (6-oz.) pieces of Pacific halibut
Salt and pepper, to taste
1 Tbsp. extra-virgin olive oil

Spinach:
1 Tbsp. extra-virgin olive oil
1 clove garlic, minced
4 cups spinach
1 Tbsp. Sunkist Almond Accents Original
   Oven Roasted Sliced Almonds

Other sides:
2 cups Uncle Ben's Long Grain & Wild Rice,
   cooked
1 lemon, cut into 8 wedges

1. For the fish: Season fillets as desired. Heat the oil in a large skillet over medium heat; add the fish and cook for 4 minutes on each side. Keep warm while you prepare the spinach.

2. For the spinach: Heat the oil and garlic in a medium skillet. When the garlic is fragrant, add the spinach and toss with tongs to wilt. Once wilted, remove from heat and garnish with sliced almonds.

3. Serve fish over a bed of rice with spinach and lemon wedges.

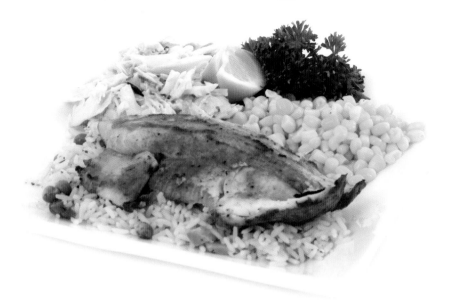

BELLY BAD

S/C Value = 7/4

BELLY GOOD

S/C Value = 1/2

Denny's Lemon Pepper Grilled Tilapia

This meal is one of the healthiest at Denny's, but it still knocks out more than half of your daily carb servings and 7 grams of sugar.

Lemon Pepper Tilapia Do-Over:

Look for wild-caught instead of farm-raised tilapia; the latter has higher levels of omega-6 fatty acids, which you already get enough of from other food sources.

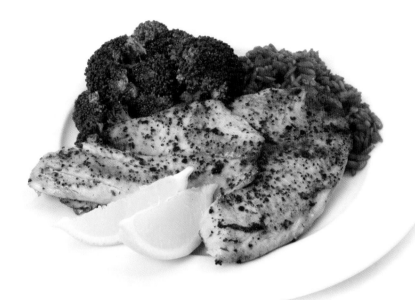

Golden Grilled Tilapia

Serves 4

Fish:
4 (6-oz.) tilapia fillets
⅓ cup white wine
1 garlic clove, minced
Salt and pepper, to taste

Broccoli:
2 cups broccoli florets
2 Tbsp. butter

Other sides:
2 cups Uncle Ben's Country Inn Mexican
   Fiesta Rice, cooked
1 lemon, cut into 8 wedges

1. For the fish: Preheat grill to medium. Place the fillets in a shallow bowl. Stir together the wine and garlic and pour over the fish. Marinate for 30 minutes, turning occasionally. Remove the fish and discard the marinade. Pat the fish dry with paper towels and season to taste. Place the fillets on a hot, well-oiled grill and cook for 2–3 minutes per side. **Note:** When grilling fish, be sure that the grate is very clean and well oiled.

2. For the broccoli: Steam the florets for 6–7 minutes; remove from heat and toss with butter.

3. Serve fish over a bed of rice with buttered broccoli and lemon wedges.

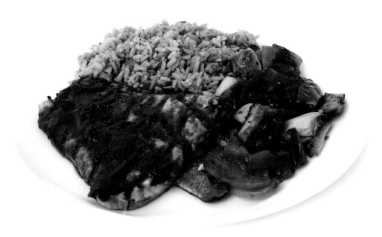

BELLY BAD

S/C Value = 20/3

BELLY GOOD

S/C Value = 2/2

Uno Chicago Grill Grilled BBQ Salmon

Fish with rice and veggies is usually a healthy dish— this one, however, tallies up a 20/3 S/C Value, which is 5 more grams of sugar than you should have all day.

BBQ Salmon Do-Over:

Cold-water fish like salmon are higher in omega-3 fatty acids than warm-water fish are. Omega-3s reduce inflammation, lower cholesterol, and improve brain function.

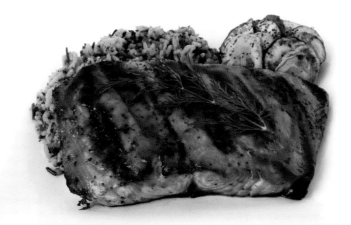

Tangy BBQ Salmon

Serves 4

Fish:
4 (6-oz.) wild-caught Atlantic salmon
    center-cut fillets
1 Tbsp. Old Bay Seasoning
½ cup Scott's Barbecue Sauce
Fresh dill sprigs, for garnish

Squash:
1 Tbsp. extra-virgin olive oil
2 garlic cloves, minced
1 cup sliced summer squash
1 cup sliced zucchini
¼ cup white wine

Other sides:
2 cups Uncle Ben's Long Grain &
    Wild Rice, cooked

1. For the salmon: Preheat grill to medium. Season the fillets with Old Bay and place on a hot, well-oiled grill. Cook for 4 minutes; turn and brush liberally with barbecue sauce. Cook for 5 minutes more; turn and brush with sauce, then turn once more and brush with sauce again. The fish is cooked when it flakes easily with a fork—do not overcook.

2. For the squash: Heat the oil and garlic in a medium skillet over medium heat. When the garlic is fragrant, add the squash and zucchini; sauté for about 7–8 minutes. Add the wine and simmer until the liquid has almost evaporated.

3. Serve the fish over a bed of rice with the sautéed squash.

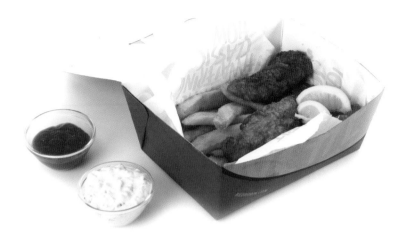

BELLY BAD

S/C Value = 4/4

BELLY GOOD

S/C Value = 1/2

Red Robin Arctic Cod Fish & Chips

Lurking inside this dish are nearly 2,800 milligrams of sodium—keep in mind that excess sodium increases the risk of hypertension and high blood pressure, which can lead to stroke or heart attack.

Fish & Chips Do-Over:

Haddock and cod are types of white fish with mild flavor, but both pack a lot of protein—a 3-oz. piece has more than 20 grams.

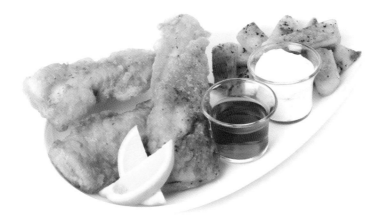

Crispy Fish & Chips

Serves 4

Fish:
Vegetable oil for deep frying
12 (4-oz.) cod or haddock fillets
2 tsp. Old Bay Seasoning
1 cup McCormick Tempura Seafood Batter Mix
¾ cup ice water

Tartar sauce:
1 cup mayonnaise
2 Tbsp. Heinz Dill Relish
2 Tbsp. finely chopped onion
½ Tbsp. parsley

Other sides:
8 oz. Ore-Ida Steak Fries
Malt vinegar, for serving
1 lemon, cut into 8 wedges

1. For the fish: Heat the oil in a large heavy skillet or saucepan, filling no more than ⅓ full. Heat to 375° F over medium heat. Cut the fish into 1" x 4" pieces and season with Old Bay. Stir together the tempura mix with ice water until thoroughly combined. Lightly coat the fish in the seafood batter and *carefully* slide it in the hot oil in batches. Fry for 3–5 minutes or until golden brown, keeping an eye on the temperature. Remove with a slotted spoon and let rest on paper towels to drain.

2. For the tartar sauce: Stir together the listed ingredients and season with some Old Bay if desired.

3. Cook fries according to package directions.

4. Serve the fish and fries along with sides of tartar sauce, malt vinegar, and lemon wedges.

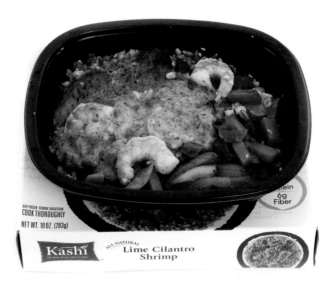

KEEP FROZEN - SERVING SUGGESTION
COOK THOROUGHLY
NET WT. 10 OZ. (283g)

Kashi ALL NATURAL Lime Cilantro Shrimp

ein
6g
Fiber

BELLY BAD

S/C Value = 8/2

Kashi Lime Cilantro Shrimp

Try Kashi Lemon Rosemary Chicken instead; with just 1 gram of sugar and 45 grams of carbs, it has a 1/3 Value—it's a bit high on carbs, but it also includes 5 grams of fiber.

BELLY GOOD

S/C Value = 3/2

Cilantro Shrimp Do-Over:

Eating shrimp can increase LDL cholesterol slightly, but it also increases levels of good cholesterol (HDL), enough so that it counteracts the slightly negative effect.

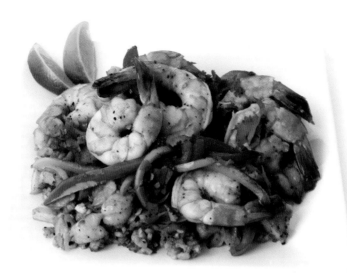

Pepper Fiesta Shrimp

Serves 4

Shrimp:
2 Tbsp. extra-virgin olive oil
1 small jalapeño, seeded and diced
3 garlic cloves, minced
1½ lbs. frozen, uncooked medium shrimp;
    thawed and peeled
½ cup sliced red bell pepper
½ cup sliced green bell pepper
½ cup sliced yellow bell pepper
2 Tbsp. chopped cilantro

Other sides:
2 cups Uncle Ben's Country Inn Mexican
    Fiesta Rice, cooked
1 lime, cut into 8 wedges

1. Heat a sauté pan to medium heat and add the oil, jalapeño, and garlic. When the garlic is fragrant, add the shrimp and sauté for 2 minutes. Add the bell peppers and sauté for 3 minutes or until the shrimp are opaque and the peppers are done to your liking. Remove from heat and toss with cilantro.

2. Serve immediately over a bed of rice with lime wedges on the side.

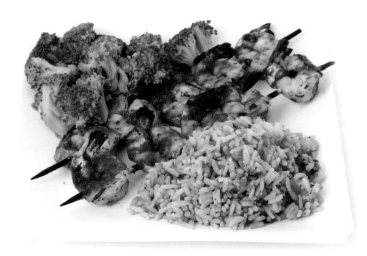

BELLY BAD

S/C Value = 14/3

Uno Chicago Grill Grilled and Skewered BBQ Shrimp

Barbecue sauce is often a main culprit in dishes like this; just 2 Tbsp. can have up to 12 grams of sugar.

BELLY GOOD

S/C Value = 2/2

BBQ Shrimp Do-Over:

Buy shrimp that have been peeled and deveined if you're in a hurry—then all you have to do is slide them onto some skewers and grill.

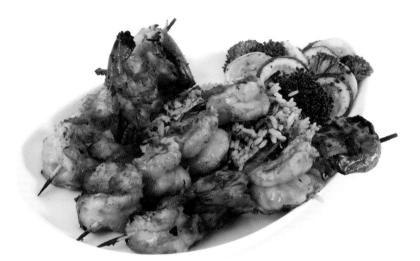

Ginger Grilled Shrimp

Serves 4

Shrimp:
12 (6") wooden skewers (soaked in water
    for at least 30 minutes)
1½ lbs. frozen, uncooked medium shrimp;
    thawed and peeled
½ cup Scott's Barbecue Sauce
1 tsp. cayenne pepper
2 cloves of garlic, minced
2 tsp. grated ginger root

Vegetables:
2 cups broccoli
1 cup summer squash, sliced into rounds
1 cup zucchini, sliced into rounds

Other sides:
2 cups Uncle Ben's Long Grain & Wild Rice, cooked

1. For the shrimp: Preheat grill to medium heat. Place 3–4 shrimp on each skewer. Mix the barbecue sauce, cayenne pepper, garlic, and ginger root together. Grill the shrimp on each side for 2 minutes; brushing barbecue sauce on the cooked side. After both sides have been coated with sauce, cook 1 minute more on each side.

2. For the vegetables: Steam for about 8 minutes; season to taste.

3. Serve shrimp skewers over a bed of rice, with a side of vegetables.

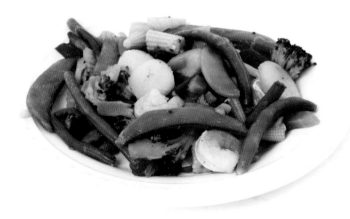

BELLY BAD

S/C Value = 20/2

Contessa Shrimp Stir-Fry

Is 189 grams of sugar a day really standard daily consumption? It's easy to see how this can happen when this dish, plus a soda = 59 grams. Two more similar meals a day, plus ice cream for dessert = more than 200 grams of sugar.

BELLY GOOD

S/C Value = 5/2

Shrimp Stir-Fry Do-Over:

Shrimp are low in calories and fat and an excellent source of protein. They're also a great source of vitamin B_{12}, which helps protect blood-vessel walls.

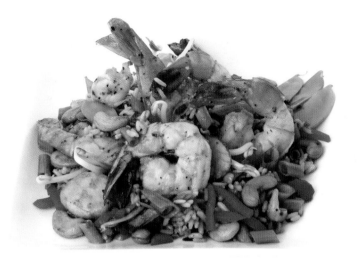

Sultry Shrimp Stir-Fry

Serves 4

Shrimp:
2 Tbsp. vegetable oil
1½ lbs. frozen, uncooked medium shrimp;
    thawed and peeled
2 garlic cloves, chopped
1 tsp. red pepper flakes
½ cup water chestnuts
½ cup snow peas
1 cup soybean sprouts
½ cup red pepper, sliced
2 packets stevia
2 tsp. toasted sesame oil
¼ cup soy sauce
2 Tbsp. balsamic vinegar
¼ cup green onion, sliced
⅓ cup cashews, raw

Other sides:
2 cups Uncle Ben's Long Grain & Wild Rice, cooked

1. Heat a large skillet over medium-high heat; add the vegetable oil. When the oil is shimmering, add the shrimp, garlic, and red pepper flakes; stir-fry for 1 minute. Add the vegetables and stir-fry for 6–8 minutes. Add the sprouts and pepper and cook for an additional 5–7 minutes. Stir together the stevia, sesame oil, soy sauce, and vinegar. Pour into the pan and cook until the shrimp is opaque and the vegetables are done to your liking. Remove from heat and stir in the green onions and cashews, reserving some of each for garnish.

2. Garnish the shrimp mixture with green onions and cashews and serve immediately over cooked rice.

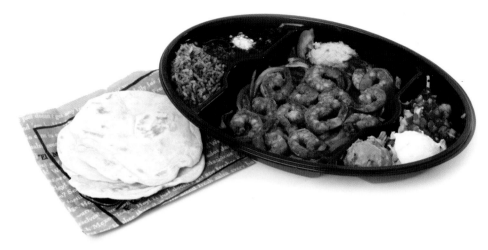

BELLY BAD

S/C Value = 21/9

BELLY GOOD

S/C Value = 5/2

Chevys Juicy Achiote Shrimp Sizzling Fajitas

Want high blood pressure?
Then eat this meal,
which has more than 5,500
milligrams of sodium.
Plus, with nearly 2,000 calories
and 21 grams of sugar,
you'll add belly fat, too.

Shrimp Fajitas Do-Over:

Having this dish
with black beans adds
5 grams of fiber.
We used Progresso canned
black beans, which have
just a few ingredients
and great flavor.

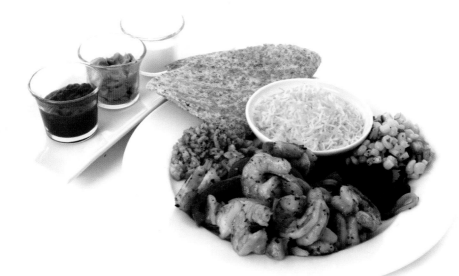

Jumbo Shrimp Fajitas

Serves 4

Fajitas:
2 Tbsp. vegetable oil
3 garlic cloves, minced
1½ lbs. frozen, uncooked medium shrimp; thawed and peeled
½ cup sliced onion
½ cup sliced red bell pepper
½ cup sliced green bell pepper
1 tsp. paprika
1 tsp. chili powder

Other sides:
½ cup canned Progresso Black Beans, drained
½ cup corn
4 La Tortilla Factory Organic Wheat Tortillas, Low Fat, Carb Cutting
½ cup Uncle Ben's Country Inn Mexican Fiesta Rice, cooked
1 cup shredded Mexican-blend cheese
4 Tbsp. Wholly Guacamole
4 Tbsp. sour cream
8 Tbsp. La Victoria Salsa Suprema
2 Tbsp. chopped cilantro, for garnish

1. Heat a large skillet to medium to high heat; add the oil and garlic. When the garlic is fragrant, add the shrimp and sauté for 1 minute. Add the onions, peppers, and spices; sauté for 3–4 minutes or until the shrimp is opaque and the vegetables are done to your liking.

2. Heat the beans and corn separately and warm the tortillas over a gas flame or in a pan. Serve the fajita mixture, beans, rice, corn, cheese, and tortillas with sides of guacamole, sour cream, and salsa. Garnish with cilantro.

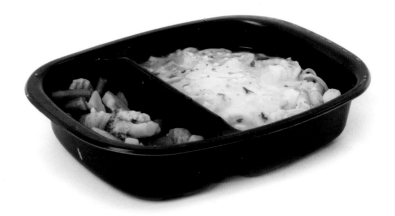

BELLY BAD

S/C Value = 5/3

Claim Jumper Shrimp Scampi

This dish just misses the cut, but if you want to lose belly fat and feel healthy and energized, every choice you make matters—so stick to dishes with a 5/2 Value or under per meal.

BELLY GOOD

S/C Value = 3/2

Shrimp Scampi Do-Over:

This dish is loaded with antioxidant- and flavor-rich garlic. It's a savory Italian meal with an S/C Value of just 3/2.

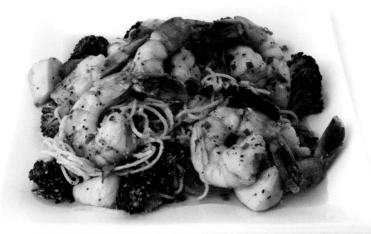

Buttered Shrimp Scampi

Serves 4

4 oz. angel-hair pasta
2 Tbsp. extra-virgin olive oil, divided use
5 Tbsp. cold butter, divided use
1 cup chopped summer squash
1 cup chopped broccoli florets
1 cup sliced carrots
2 Tbsp. chopped parsley
3 garlic cloves, minced
1½ lbs. frozen, uncooked medium shrimp;
    thawed and peeled
½ cup white wine
2 Tbsp. finely chopped chives

1. Cook the pasta according to package directions; drain and set aside. Heat 1 Tbsp. of the olive oil and 1 Tbsp. of the butter in a large skillet over medium heat. When the butter has melted, sauté the vegetables until tender, about 8 minutes. Transfer to a bowl and toss with parsley; set aside.

2. In the same skillet, heat 1 Tbsp. of the olive oil, 1 Tbsp. of the butter, and the garlic over medium heat until the butter is melted and the garlic is fragrant. Sauté the shrimp for 2 minutes; remove and place on a plate. Turn the heat to medium high; add the wine and let reduce by half. Whisk in the remaining butter, 1 Tbsp. at a time, to incorporate into the wine reduction. Add the shrimp and vegetables back into the pan; simmer until the shrimp is opaque and the vegetables are heated through.

3. Spoon the shrimp and vegetables with sauce over the pasta. Garnish with chopped chives and serve.

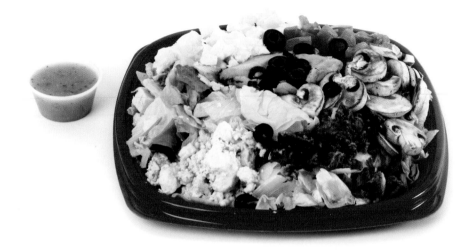

BELLY BAD

S/C Value = 8/2

Ruby's Diner Cobb Salad

With several ingredients, it's easy for a Cobb salad to topple the recommended sugar amount of 5 grams per meal; this one certainly does with its 8 grams. Also, watch out for fat-free dressings, which often add excess sugar.

BELLY GOOD

S/C Value = 3/1

Cobb Salad Do-Over:

Homemade blue-cheese dressing makes this meal a winner. It's quick and easy and has no mysterious ingredients like so many store-bought brands do.

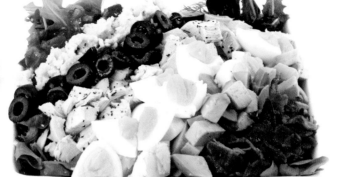

Lovely Cobb Salad

Serves 4

Salad:
½ head romaine lettuce, chopped
1 head red-leaf lettuce, chopped
12 strips of bacon, cooked and chopped
4 hard-boiled eggs, chopped
1 avocado, diced
2 cups diced cooked chicken
½ cup diced tomato
1 cup sliced black olives

Blue-cheese dressing:
½ cup extra-virgin olive oil
3 Tbsp. red-wine vinegar
1 tsp. Dijon mustard
⅓ cup blue-cheese crumbles
1 tsp. chopped shallots
Salt and pepper, to taste

1. For the salad: Toss chopped lettuces together and divide evenly among 4 serving plates. Arrange remaining ingredients on the lettuce as desired.

2. For the dressing: Mix all listed ingredients in a blender and pulse until smooth; season to taste with salt and pepper.

3. Serve each salad with a side of dressing.

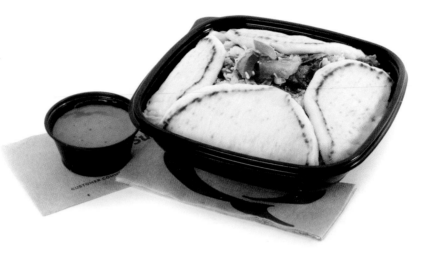

BELLY BAD

S/C Value = 38/5

Quiznos Raspberry Chipotle Chicken Flatbread Chopped Salad

Most of this salad's shocking sugar value comes from the Raspberry Chipotle Dressing—a single serving has 33 grams of sugar. Pay attention to dressings and sauces; they can be sneaky.

BELLY GOOD

S/C Value = 4/1

Chopped Salad Do-Over:

Carrots, cucumber, and tomatoes add vitamins A, K, and C to this salad. Toast the pitas for a little extra crunch.

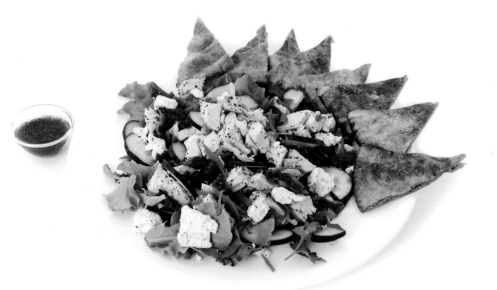

Bacon & Feta Chicken Salad

Serves 4

Salad:
½ head romaine lettuce, chopped
1 head red-leaf lettuce, chopped
2 large chicken breasts, cooked and diced
½ cup grated carrots
½ English cucumber, peeled, seeded, and diced
12 strips of bacon, cooked and crumbled
½ cup diced tomato
½ cup crumbled feta cheese

Tangy dressing:
⅓ cup extra-virgin olive oil
2 Tbsp. red-wine vinegar
1 tsp. Dijon mustard
Salt and pepper, to taste

Other sides:
2 (6") Sara Lee Mr. Pita Whole Wheat Pita
    Breads, toasted and cut into wedges

1. For the salad: Arrange lettuces on 4 chilled salad plates. Top with remaining ingredients.

2. For the dressing: Whisk together the vinegar and mustard. Keep whisking while slowly pouring in the oil. Season to taste with salt and pepper.

3. Serve each salad with a side of dressing and some toasted pita wedges.

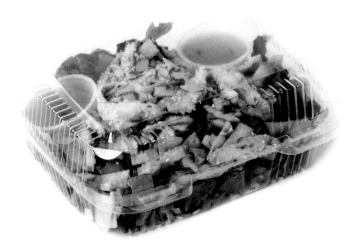

BELLY BAD

S/C Value = 11/2

BELLY GOOD

S/C Value = 3/1

Panera Bread Asian Sesame Chicken Salad

The "reduced sugar" dressing with this salad actually has 4 grams of it—which is the equivalent of dumping a teaspoon of sugar on your salad.

Asian Sesame Chicken Salad Do-Over:

Out of all of the nuts and seeds, sesame seeds have the highest content of phytosterols, a cholesterol-lowering, immune-boosting compound.

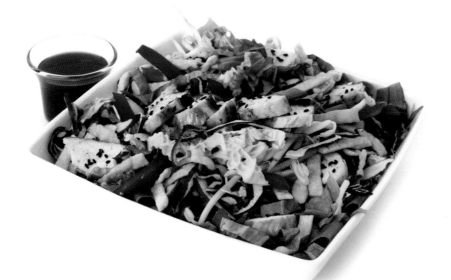

Crunchy Sesame Chicken Salad

Serves 4

Salad:
3 cups romaine lettuce, shredded
2 cups Napa cabbage, shredded
½ cup red cabbage, shredded
2 large chicken breasts, cooked and sliced
1 cup sliced red bell pepper
1 cup soybean sprouts
8 Tbsp. Fresh Gourmet Authentic Wonton Strips
¼ cup Planters Recipe Ready Slivered Almonds
¼ cup thinly sliced green onion, for garnish
1 Tbsp. black sesame seeds, for garnish

Asian dressing:
3 Tbsp. Eden Organic Brown Rice Vinegar
2 Tbsp. xylitol
2 tsp. soy sauce
1 Tbsp. sesame oil
¼ cup vegetable oil

1. For the salad: Toss the lettuce and cabbages together and divide evenly among 4 chilled salad plates. Arrange the remaining ingredients on the greens, except for the green onions and sesame seeds, as desired.

2. For the dressing: Whisk all of the listed ingredients together and season to taste.

3. Garnish each salad with green onions and sesame seeds, and serve with a side of dressing.

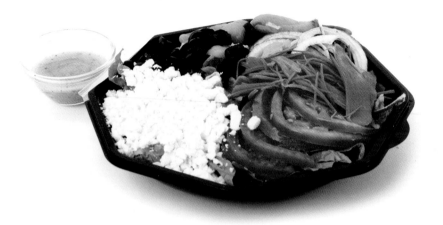

BELLY BAD

S/C Value = 7/1

BELLY GOOD

S/C Value = 5/2

Schlotzsky's Greek Salad

This salad is low in carbs but has 7 grams of sugar—that's 2 more than you should have per meal if you want to lose belly fat and keep your immune system strong.

Greek Salad Do-Over:

Make quick and easy croutons using Food for Life Ezekiel 4:9 bread and you've added no extra sugar to this salad. Bake a big batch of them and store in a Ziploc bag.

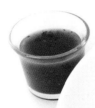
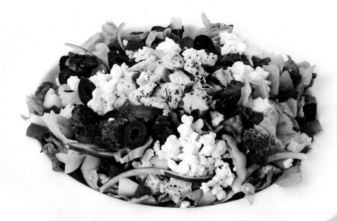

Garden Fresh Greek Salad

Serves 4

Salad:
1 head romaine lettuce, chopped
2 cups shredded rotisserie chicken (recommended: Kirkland brand)
4 slices red onion, separated
1 cup English cucumber, thinly sliced
¾ cup crumbled feta cheese
¼ cup pitted Kalamata olives
1 cup diced tomato
4 pepperoncinis, sliced
½ tsp. dried oregano

Croutons:
4 slices Food for Life Ezekiel 4:9 Sprouted 100% Whole Grain Bread, cut into cubes
2 Tbsp. butter, melted
½ tsp. dried oregano
1 clove garlic, minced

Red-wine vinaigrette:
⅓ cup extra-virgin olive oil
¼ cup red-wine vinegar
1 tsp. dried oregano

1. For the salad: Divide the lettuce evenly among 4 chilled salad plates. Arrange the remaining ingredients on the greens.

2. For the croutons: Preheat oven to 350° F. Stir together the melted butter, oregano, and garlic in a large bowl. Add the bread crumbs and toss. Spread evenly on a baking sheet and toast in a preheated oven for 10–15 minutes or until golden and crisp.

3. For the vinaigrette: Whisk the oil, vinegar, and oregano together and season to taste.

4. Top each salad with croutons and serve with a side of dressing.

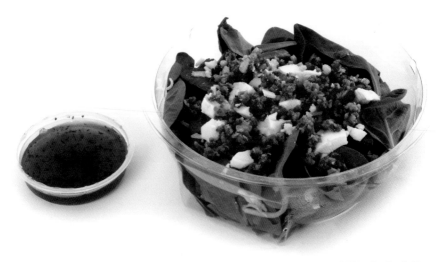

BELLY BAD

S/C Value = 8/1

Ready Pac Bistro Spinach Bacon Salad

The honey bacon dressing adds most of the sugar to this salad; it's also made with corn syrup and has sodium nitrite—two things I recommend avoiding when you can.

BELLY GOOD

S/C Value = 0/1

Spinach Bacon Salad Do-Over:

Spinach has 200% of the recommended amount of vitamin K, which helps maintain bone health and aids in blood clotting.

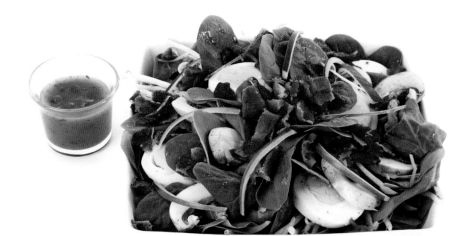

Summer Spinach Salad

Serves 4

Salad:
12 oz. baby spinach
4 slices red onion
1 cup sliced button mushrooms
¼ cup bean sprouts
2 hard-boiled eggs, sliced
4 strips of bacon, cooked and chopped

Warm vinaigrette:
½ cup extra-virgin olive oil
2 Tbsp. red-wine vinegar
3 Tbsp. Nature's Hollow Sugar Free Ketchup
½ Tbsp. dehydrated onion flakes

1. For the salad: Divide the spinach evenly among 4 serving plates. Arrange the remaining ingredients on the greens.

2. For the dressing: Mix all listed ingredients in a small saucepan and warm over low heat; whisk well and season to taste.

3. Serve each salad with a side of dressing.

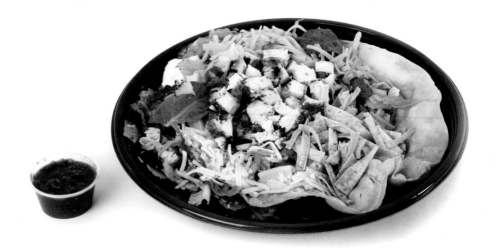

BELLY BAD

S/C Value = 11/6

Chevys Tostada Salad with Chicken

The tostada "bowl" of this salad will wipe out all of your carbs for the day. Unless you plan on eating just protein for the rest of the day, I suggest a smarter choice.

BELLY GOOD

S/C Value = 2/2

Tostada Salad with Chicken Do-Over:

La Tortilla Factory's brand of tortillas make the "bowl" here. This way, you can enjoy a traditional taco salad for just a 2/2 on the S/C Value.

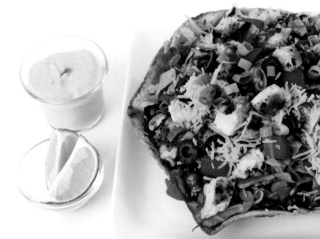

Tantalizing Taco Salad

Serves 4

Salad:
4 La Tortilla Factory Smart & Delicious Low Fat
    Tortillas
2 Tbsp. extra-virgin olive oil
1 cup shredded romaine lettuce
1 cup shredded green-leaf lettuce
3 cups chopped baby spinach
2 cups chopped rotisserie chicken (recommended:
    Kirkland brand)
½ cup canned Progresso Black Beans, drained
1 cup shredded cheddar cheese
½ cup sliced black olives
½ cup diced tomatoes
4 green onions, thinly sliced

Salsa crema dressing:
½ cup La Victoria Salsa Suprema
¼ cup mayonnaise
¼ cup sour cream
1 clove garlic, minced
½ lime, juiced

Other sides:
1 lime, cut into 8 wedges

1. For the salad: Preheat oven to 400° F. Brush
the tortillas with olive oil on both sides. Press into
4 oven-safe bowls (the size you want your tortilla
bowl to be) and set on a cookie sheet. Bake for
10–15 minutes or until crispy. Remove the tortilla
bowls from the oven and let cool. Toss the lettuces and spinach together and divide among
the cooled tortilla bowls. Top with the remaining
ingredients.

2. For the dressing: Combine all listed ingredients;
mix thoroughly and season to taste.

3. Serve taco salad with lime wedges and a side of
dressing.

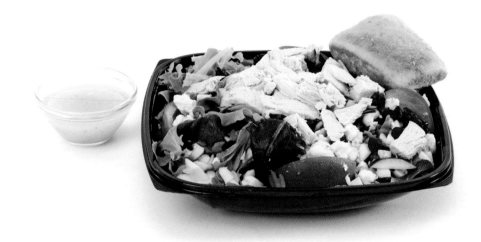

BELLY BAD

S/C Value = 26/3

Boston Market Market Chopped Salad with Chicken

Craisins (dried cranberries) have almost 30 grams of sugar in ⅓ cup—that means even when they're sprinkled on as they are here, they can do some damage.

BELLY GOOD

S/C Value = 3/1

Chopped Salad Do-Over:

Both spinach and arugula are excellent sources of vitamins A and C and folic acid. Top with antioxidant-rich raspberries and cholesterol-lowering pecans, and you've got a nutritional powerhouse.

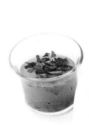

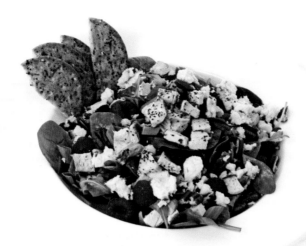

Pecan Delight Chopped Salad

Serves 4

Salad:
2 large chicken breasts, cooked and diced
1 bag (6 oz.) arugula, chopped
1 bag (6 oz.) baby spinach, chopped
½ cup raspberries
¼ cup chopped pecans
¼ cup Gorgonzola or goat cheese, crumbled

Dressing:
½ cup extra-virgin olive oil
3 tsp. red-wine vinegar
1 packet stevia
1 tsp. Dijon mustard
1 tsp. chopped shallot

Other sides:
8 Milton's Everything Multi-Grain Crackers

1. For the salad: Toss together the chopped arugula and spinach and divide evenly among 4 chilled salad bowls. Top with the remaining ingredients.

2. For the dressing: Whisk all listed ingredients until incorporated and season to taste.

3. Serve each salad with 2 crackers and a side of dressing.

Website Product Finder

Many of the following products are available for sale at **TheBellyFatCure.com**, or you can find more information by visiting the Websites listed below:

Almond Breeze Unsweetened Almond Milk: **bluediamond.com**

Amazing Grass Green SuperFood Chocolate Drink Powder: **amazinggrass.com**

Arrowhead Mills Organic Soy Flour: **arrowheadmills.com**

Barlean's Omega Swirl: **barleans.com**

Bob's Red Mill Egg Replacer: **bobsredmill.com**

Cascadian Farm Hash Browns: **cascadianfarm.com**

Clemmy's Ice Cream: **clemmysicecream.com**

DeLallo Organic Whole Wheat Pasta: **delallo.com**

Doctor's CarbRite Diet Bars: **carbritediet.com**

El Burrito Soyrizo and SoyTaco: **elburrito.com**

Ener-G Foods Light Brown Rice Loaf: **ener-g.com**

FAGE Yogurt: **fageusa.com**

Follow Your Heart Vegenaise & Vegan Gourmet Cheese Alternatives: **followyourheart.com**

Food for Life Ezekiel 4:9 Products: **foodforlife.com**

Hershey's Sugar Free Chocolate Chips: **hersheys.com**

It's All Good Meat-free Products: **itsallgoodfoods.com**

Jay Robb Whey Protein: **jayrobb.com**

Jennies Unsweetened Coconut Macaroons: **macaroonking.com**

Joseph's Sugar-Free Cookies & Maple Syrup: **josephslitecookies.com**

Judy's Candy Company Sugar Free Caramels & Peanut Brittle: **judyscandy.com**

La Tortilla Factory: **latortillafactory.com**

LowCarb Specialties, Inc. ChocoPerfection: **lowcarbspecialties.com**

Morningstar Farms Veggie Patties: **morningstarfarms.com**

Nature's Hollow Sugar Free Ketchup, Preserves & Syrups: **probstfarms.com**

Nature's Plus Source of Life Red and Bright Lightning: **naturesplus.com**

Oroweat Light 100% Whole Wheat Bread & Hot Dog Buns: **oroweat.com**

Perfectly Sweet Licorice & Cinna Cubs: **perfectlysweet.com**

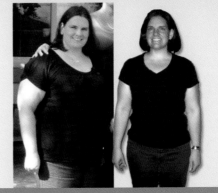

Pirate's Booty: **piratesbooty.com**

PureVia: **purevia.com**

Rice Expressions: **riceandrecipes.com**

Rosetto All-Natural Whole Wheat Cheese
Ravioli: **rosetto.com**

Rudi's Organic Bakery Whole Grain Breads:
rudisbakery.com

Scott's Barbecue Sauce:
scottsbarbecuesauce.com

Seeds of Change Pasta Sauce:
seedsofchangefoods.com

Seelect Teas' Organic Caramel Syrup:
seelecttea.com

Simply Potatoes: **simplypotatoes.com**

Stevia SweetLeaf Sweetener: **sweetleaf.com**

Truvia: **truvia.com**

Tumaro's Gourmet Tortillas: **tumaros.com**

Ultima Replenisher Drinks: **ultimareplenisher
.com**

U.S. Mills Uncle Sam Cereal: **usmillsllc.com**

Vega Whole Food Health Optimizer:
sequelnaturals.com/vega

Vitalicious VitaMuffins and VitaTops:
vitalicious.com

Wholly Guacamole: **whollyguac.com**

Xlear, Inc. SparX Candy: **xlear.com**

Xlear, Inc. Spry Gum and Mints: **xlear.com**

Xlear, Inc. Xylitol Products: **xlear.com**

Zevia Soda: **zevia.com**

Mary Lynne lost 50 pounds

Age: 32
Height: 5'2"
Pounds Lost: 50
Belly Inches Lost: 9.5

"I've always struggled with my weight and confidence, but with this program, I was finally empowered to take control. The program was so easy to follow, and I could still eat all of the foods I really like. Since losing weight, I have more confidence, more energy, more joy, more happiness, more clothes, and more dates! I've even inspired others to take control of their health and start losing weight. It's a great feeling knowing that not only did I make a difference in my own life, but in others' lives as well. I now look forward to what the future has in store for me."

BEST TIP FOR SUCCESS:

"The key to eating out is sticking to foods for which you know the S/C value and asking the chef to limit anything that's high in sugar. Restaurants are very accommodating to these requests, so don't be afraid to ask."

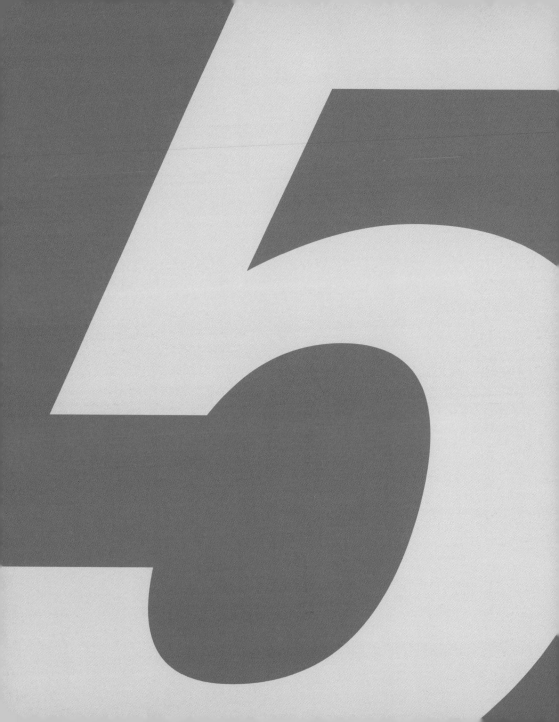

5 Carb Swap
Products

In addition to the Belly Good meals in the last chapter, you need to know what to fill your pantry and refrigerator with in order to truly make the Belly Fat Cure an everyday lifestyle. The following 17 product categories feature, by brand name, the most popular foods and items you need to stock in your kitchen, along with their S/C Values. I've included sweeteners, breads, pastas, fruits and vegetables, condiments, and several more.

Focus on the Belly Good side of the Carb Swaps for my recommended products for the Belly Fat Cure. Be sure to check out the products and brands I call attention to along the bottom of the page. These items have also been awarded our official seal of approval because of their exceptional adherence to the S/C Value, and because they're extraordinarily great-tasting products. For your reference, I've also included the Belly Bad foods and products I urge you to avoid as much as possible. Some items are too high in sugar if you want to lose belly fat and achieve your best health; others contain artificial sweeteners, which I recommend you stay away from if you can.

Review the Belly Good foods before you head to the grocery store, or take the book with you so that you can easily spot the items you're looking for. Either way, these Carb Swap products will be an essential tool for your success. Start shopping today!

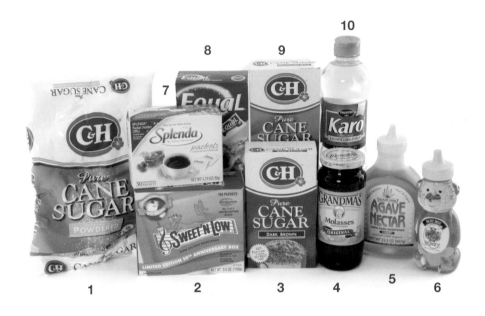

BELLY BAD

1. C&H Pure Cane Powdered Sugar (¼ cup): 29/2. 2. Sweet'N Low (1 pink packet): 0/0. 3. C&H Pure Cane Dark Brown Sugar (1 tsp.): 4/0. 4. Grandma's Original Molasses (1 Tbsp.): 10/1. 5. Madhava Agave Nectar (1 Tbsp.): 15/1. 6. Busy Bee Honey (1 Tbsp.): 16/1. 7. Splenda (1 yellow packet): 0/0. 8. Equal (1 blue packet): 0/0. 9. C & H Pure Cane Granulated Sugar (1 tsp.): 4/0. 10. Karo Light Corn Syrup (2 Tbsp.): 10/2.

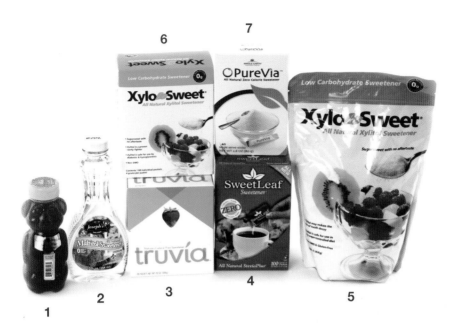

BELLY GOOD

1. Nature's Hollow Tastes Like Honey (1 Tbsp.): 0/1. 2. Joseph's Maltitol Sweetener (¼ cup): 0/1
3. Truvia (1 packet): 0/0. 4. SweetLeaf Sweetener All Natural SteviaPlus (1 packet): 0/0. 5. Xlear, Inc.
XyloSweet (1 tsp.): 0/0. 6. Xlear, Inc. XyloSweet (1 packet): 0/0. 7. PureVia (1 stick): 0/0.

**The Belly Fat Cure Seal of Approval has been
awarded to all products above.**

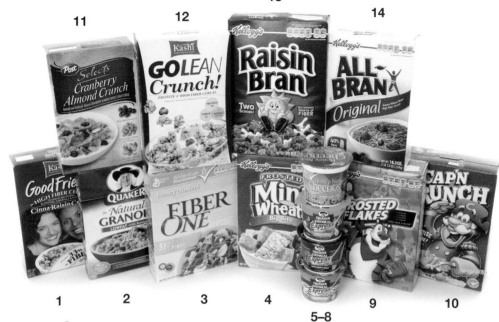

BELLY BAD

1. Kashi Good Friends Cinna-Raisin Crunch (1 cup): 13/3. 2. Quaker Natural Granola Lowfat with Raisins (⅔ cup): 18/3. 3. General Mills Fiber One Honey Clusters (1 cup): 6/3. 4. Kellogg's Frosted Mini-Wheats Big Bite (5 biscuits): 10/3. 5. General Mills Honey Nut Cheerios (1 container): 17/3. 6. Quaker Oatmeal Express Baked Apple (1 container): 19/3. 7. Quaker Oatmeal Express Golden Brown Sugar (1 container): 18/3. 8. Quaker Oatmeal Express Cinnamon Roll (1 container): 17/3. 9. Kellogg's Frosted Flakes (¾ cup): 11/2. 10. Quaker Cap'n Crunch (¾ cup): 12/2. 11. Post Selects Cranberry Almond Crunch (¾ cup): 13/2. 12. Kashi GoLean Crunch! (1 cup): 13/2. 13. Kellogg's Raisin Bran (1 cup): 19/3. 14. Kellogg's All-Bran (½ cup): 6/2.

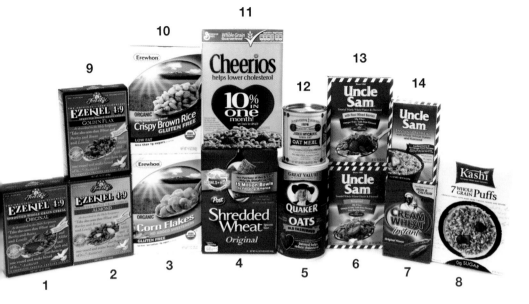

9
10
11
12
13
14
1
2
3
4
5
6
7
8

BELLY GOOD

1. Food for Life Ezekiel 4:9 Original Cereal (½ cup): 0/2. 2. Food for Life Ezekiel 4:9 Almond Cereal (½ cup): 0/2. 3. U.S. Mills Erewhon Corn Flakes (1 cup): 0/2. 4. Post Shredded Wheat (1 cup): 0/2. 5. Old Fashioned Quaker Oats (½ cup): 1/2. 6. U.S. Mills Uncle Sam Cereal Original (3/4 cup): 0/2. 7. B&G Instant Cream of Wheat (1 packet): 0/1. 8. Kashi 7 Whole Grain Puffs (1 cup): 0/1. 9. Food for Life Ezekiel 4:9 Golden Flax Cereal (½ cup): 0/2. 10. U.S. Mills Erewhon Crispy Brown Rice Gluten Free (1 cup): 0/2. 11. General Mills Cheerios (1 cup) 1/1. 12. McCann's Steel-Cut Irish Oatmeal (¼ cup): 0/2. 13. U.S. Mills Uncle Sam Cereal with Mixed Berries (3/4 cup): 2/2. 14. U.S. Mills Uncle Sam Instant Oatmeal (1 packet): 0/2.

The Belly Fat Cure Seal of Approval has been awarded to all U.S. Mills (Uncle Sam and Erewhon) products above.

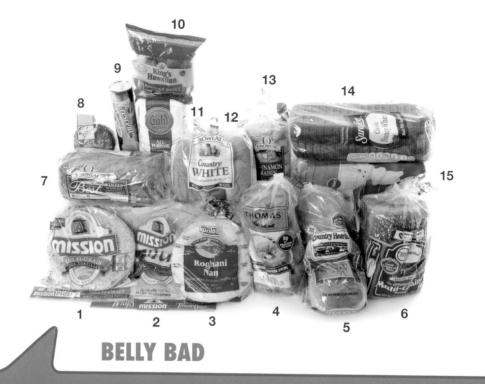

BELLY BAD

1. Mission Multi-Grain Flour Tortillas (1 tortilla): 2/2. 2. Mission Sundried Tomato Basil Wraps (1 wrap): 4/2. 3. Kontos Roghani Nan (1 pocket): 5/2. 4. Thomas' Cinnamon Raisin Swirl Bagels (1 bagel): 12/3. 5. Country Hearth Giant Onion Buns (1 bun): 7/3. 6. Milton's Healthy Multi-Grain Bread (1 slice): 5/2. 7. Oroweat Master's Best Winter Wheat Bread (1 slice): 3/1. 8. Bon Appetit Banana Nut Muffin (1 muffin): 39/4. 9. Pillsbury Big & Buttery Crescent Rolls (1 roll): 4/1. 10. King's Hawaiian Original Hawaiian Sweet Rolls (1 roll): 7/1. 11. Gold Medal All-Purpose Flour (¼ cup): 0/2. 12. Oroweat Country White Hot Dog Buns (1 bun): 6/2. 13. Oroweat Cinnamon Raisin English Muffins (1 muffin): 11/2. 14. Sara Lee Classic Honey Wheat Bread (1 slice): 3/1. 15. Pillsbury Buttermilk Bread (1 slice): 3/1.

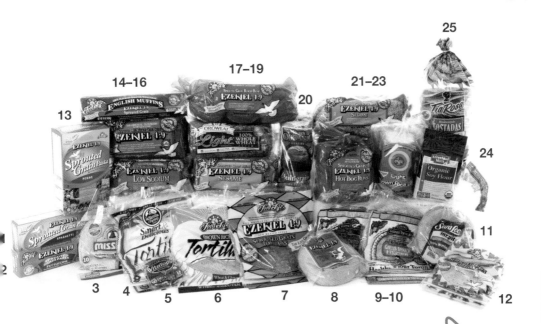

BELLY GOOD

1. Food for Life Ezekiel 4:9 Sprouted Whole Grain Pasta Spaghetti (2 oz.): 0/2. 2. Food for Life Ezekiel 4:9 Sprouted Whole Grain Pasta Fettuccine (2 oz.): 0/2. 3. Mission Yellow Corn Tortillas Super Size (1 tortilla): 2/1. 4. La Tortilla Factory Smart & Delicious Low Carb High Fiber Tortillas (1 tortilla): 1/1. 5. Vitalicious Banana Nut VitaTops (1 VitaTop): 0/2. 6. Food For Life Brown Rice Tortillas (1 tortilla): 0/2. 7. Food for Life Ezekiel 4:9 Sprouted Grain Tortillas (1 tortilla): 0/2. 8. Food for Life Ezekiel 4:9 Prophets Pocket (1 pocket): 1/2. 9. Tumaro's Sun-Dried Tomato & Basil Healthy Flour Tortillas (1 tortilla; 8-inch): 0/2. 10. Tumaro's Garden Spinach & Vegetables Healthy Flour Tortillas (1 tortilla; 8-inch): 0/2. 11. Sara Lee Mr. Pita Whole Wheat Pita (1 pocket): 1/1. 12. Food For Life Sprouted Corn Tortillas (2 tortillas): 1/2. 13. Food for Life Ezekiel 4:9 Sprouted Whole Grain Pasta Penne (2 oz.): 0/2. 14. Food for Life Ezekiel 4:9 Sprouted Grain English Muffins (1 muffin): 0/2. 15. Food for Life Ezekiel 4:9 Sprouted 100% Whole Grain Bread (1 slice): 0/1. 16. Food for Life Ezekiel 4:9 Sprouted Grain Bread Low Sodium (1 slice): 0/1. 17. Food for Life Ezekiel 4:9 Sprouted Grain Burger Buns (1 bun): 0/2. 18. Oroweat Light 100% Whole Wheat Bread (2 slices): 3/1. 19. Food for Life Ezekiel 4:9 Sprouted Grain Sesame Bread (1 slice): 0/1. 20. Rudi's Organic Bakery Multigrain Bagels (1 bagel): 3/2. 21. Food for Life Ezekiel 4:9 Sprouted Grain Burger Buns Sesame (1 bun): 0/2. 22. Food for Life Ezekiel 4:9 Sprouted Grain Hot Dog Buns (1 bun): 0/2. 23. Ener-G Foods Light Brown Rice Loaf (1 slice): 1/1. 24. Arrowhead Mills Organic Soy Flour (¼ cup): 0/1. 25. Tia Rosa Homestyle Tostadas (1 piece): 0/1.

**The Belly Fat Cure Seal of Approval has been awarded
to all Ezekiel 4:9 and Food for Life products above.**

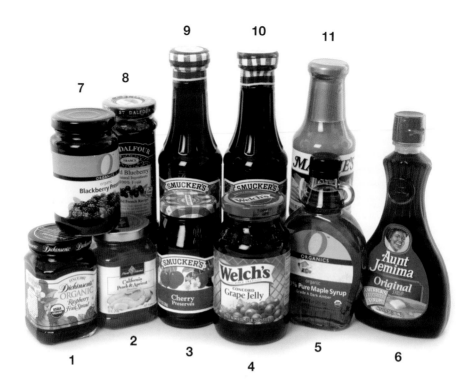

BELLY BAD

1. Dickinson's Organic Raspberry Fruit Spread (1 Tbsp.): 10/1. 2. Private Selection California Peach & Apricot Preserves (1 Tbsp.): 12/1. 3. Smucker's Cherry Preserves (1 Tbsp.): 12/1. 4. Welch's Concord Grape Jelly (1 Tbsp.): 13/1. 5. O Organics Grade A Dark Amber 100% Pure Maple Syrup (¼ cup): 50/3. 6. Aunt Jemima Original Syrup (¼ cup): 32/3. 7. O Organics Blackberry Preserve (1 Tbsp.): 12/1. 8. St. Dalfour Wild Blueberry Fruit Spread (1 Tbsp.): 13/1. 9. Smucker's Strawberry Syrup (¼ cup): 44/3. 10. Smucker's Boysenberry Syrup (¼ cup): 44/3. 11. Margie's Banana Syrup (¼ cup): 34/2.

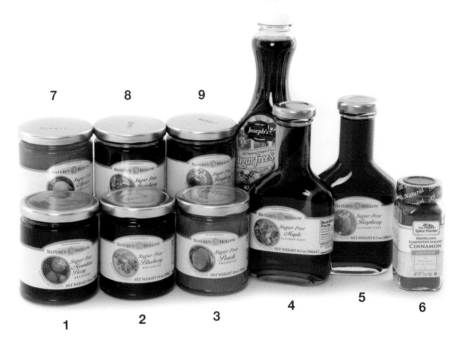

10

7   **8**   **9**

1   **2**   **3**   **4**   **5**   **6**

BELLY GOOD

1. Nature's Hollow Sugar Free Mountain Berry Preserves (1 Tbsp.): 0/1. 2. Nature's Hollow Sugar Free Blueberry Preserves (1 Tbsp): 0/1. 3. Nature's Hollow Sugar Free Peach Preserves (1 Tbsp.): 0/1. 4. Nature's Hollow Sugar Free Maple Flavored Syrup (¼ cup): 0/1. 5. Nature's Hollow Sugar Free Raspberry Flavored Syrup (¼ cup): 0/1. 6. The Spice Hunter Highland Harvested Saigon Cinnamon, Ground (1 tsp.): 0/0. 7. Nature's Hollow Sugar Free Apricot Preserves (1 Tbsp.): 0/1. 8. Nature's Hollow Sugar Free Strawberry Preserves (1 Tbsp.): 0/1. 9. Nature's Hollow Sugar Free Raspberry Preserves (1 Tbsp.): 0/1. 10. Joseph's Sugar Free Maple Syrup (¼ cup): 0/1.

**The Belly Fat Cure Seal of Approval has been awarded
to all Nature's Hollow and Joseph's products above.**

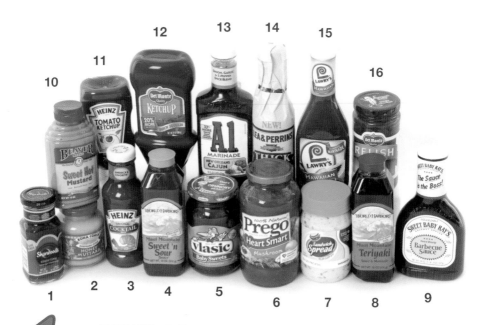

BELLY BAD

1. Sharwood's Mango Chutney (¼ cup): 39/3. 2. Kona Coast Hawaiian Style Honey Mustard (1 tsp.): 3/0. 3. Heinz Cocktail Sauce (¼ cup): 11/1. 4. World Harbors Maui Mountain Sweet 'n Sour Sauce (2 Tbsp.): 12/1. 5. Vlasic Baby Sweets (1 pickle): 9/1. 6. Prego Heart Smart Mushroom Italian Sauce (½ cup): 9/1. 7. Safeway Sandwich Spread (1 Tbsp.): 2/0. 8. World Harbors Maui Mountain Teriyaki Sauce & Marinade (2 Tbsp.): 15/1. 9. Sweet Baby Ray's Barbecue Sauce (2 Tbsp.): 16/1. 10. Beaver Brand Sweet Hot Mustard (1 tsp.): 2/0. 11. Heinz Tomato Ketchup (1 Tbsp.): 4/0. 12. Del Monte Ketchup (1 Tbsp.): 4/0. 13. A.1. New Orleans Cajun Marinade (1 Tbsp.): 5/1. 14. Lea & Perrins Thick Classic Worcestershire Sauce (2 Tbsp.): 6/1. 15. Lawry's Hawaiian Marinade (1 Tbsp.): 5/1. 16. Del Monte Sweet Relish (1 Tbsp.): 5/1.

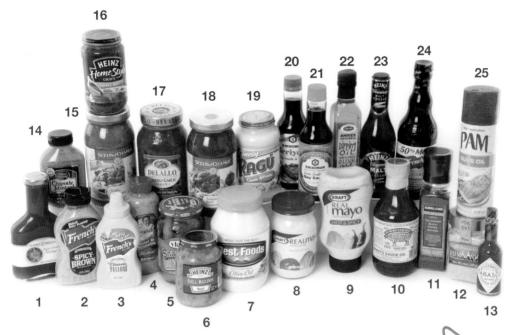

BELLY GOOD

1. Nature's Hollow Sugar Free Ketchup (1 Tbsp.): 0/1. 2. French's Spicy Brown Mustard (1 tsp.): 0/0.
3. French's Classic Yellow Mustard (1 tsp.): 0/0. 4. Emeril's Kicked Up Horseradish Mustard (1 tsp.): 0/0.
5. Vlasic Snack'mms Kosher Dill (3 pickles): 1/0. 6. Heinz Dill Relish (1 Tbsp.): 0/0. 7. Best Foods Mayonnaise Dressing with Extra Virgin Olive Oil (1 Tbsp.): 0/0. 8. Kraft Real Mayo (1 Tbsp.): 0/0. 9. Kraft Real Mayo Hot & Spicy (1 Tbsp.): 0/0. 10. Scott's Barbecue Sauce (2 Tbsp.): 0/0. 11. Kirkland Signature Tellicherry Black Pepper Grinder (¼ tsp.): 0/0. 12. Himalania Pink Salt (¼ tsp.): 0/0. 13. Tabasco Pepper Sauce (1 tsp.): 0/0. 14. Silver Springs Chipotle Mustard (1 tsp.): 0/0. 15. Seeds of Change Vodka Americano Pasta Sauce (½ cup): 1/1. 16. Heinz Savory Beef HomeStyle Gravy (¼ cup): 0/0. 17. DeLallo Roasted Garlic Pasta Sauce (½ cup): 1/1. 18. Seeds of Change Tomato Basil Genovese Pasta Sauce (½ cup): 0/1. 19. Ragú Cheesy Classic Alfredo Sauce (¼ cup): 0/0. 20. Kikkoman Teriyaki Marinade & Sauce (1 Tbsp.): 2/0. 21. Kikkoman Less Sodium Soy Sauce (1 Tbsp.): 0/0. 22. Annie's Naturals Dipping Oil (1 Tbsp.): 0/0. 23. Heinz Malt Vinegar (1 Tbsp.): 0/0. 24. French's Reduced Sodium Worcestershire Sauce (1 tsp.): 0/0. 25. Pam Olive Oil No-Stick Cooking Spray (⅓ second spray): 0/0.

**The Belly Fat Cure Seal of Approval has been awarded
to Scott's Barbecue Sauce and Nature's Hollow Sugar Free Ketchup.**

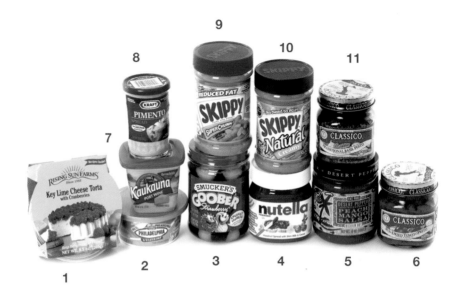

BELLY BAD

1. Rising Sun Farms Key Lime Cheese Torta (1 oz.): 7/1. 2. Kraft Philadelphia Garden Vegetable Soft Cream Cheese (2 Tbsp.): 2/0. 3. Smucker's Goober PB & J Strawberry (3 Tbsp.): 21/2. 4. Ferrero Nutella (2 Tbsp.): 21/2. 5. Desert Pepper Trading Company Peach Mango Salsa (2 Tbsp.): 3/0. 6. Classico Sun-Dried Tomato Pesto (¼ cup): 5/1. 7. Kaukauna Port Wine Spreadable Cheese (2 Tbsp.): 4/0. 8. Kraft Pimento Spread (2 Tbsp.): 3/0. 9. Skippy Reduced Fat Super Chunk (2 Tbsp.): 4/1. 10. Skippy Natural Creamy (2 Tbsp.): 3/1. 11. Classico Traditional Basil Pesto (¼ cup): 2/1.

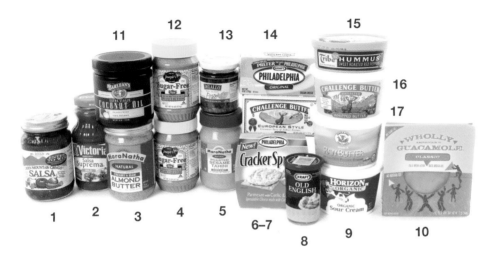

11 12 13 14 15 16 17

1 2 3 4 5 6–7 8 9 10

BELLY GOOD

1. Green Mountain Gringo Salsa (2 Tbsp.): 0/0. 2. La Victoria Salsa Suprema (2 Tbsp.): 1/0. 3. MaraNatha Natural Almond Butter Creamy & Raw (2 Tbsp.): 2/1. 4. Joseph's Sugar-Free Creamy Valencia Peanut Butter (2 Tbsp): 0/1. 5. MaraNatha Natural Sesame Tahini Creamy & Roasted (2 Tbsp.): 0/1. 6. Kraft Philadelphia Cracker Spread Parmesan with Garlic & Herbs (2 Tbsp.): 0/0. 7. Challenge Butter European Style, stick (1 Tbsp.): 0/0. 8. Kraft Old English Cheese Spread (2 Tbsp.): 0/0. 9. Horizon Organic Sour Cream (2 Tbsp.): 1/0. 10. Wholly Guacamole (2 Tbsp.): 0/0. 11. Barlean's Extra Virgin Coconut Oil (1 Tbsp.): 0/0. 12. Joseph's Sugar-Free Crunchy Valencia Peanut Butter (2 Tbsp): 0/1. 13. DeLallo Pesto (1 Tbsp.): 0/0. 14. Kraft Philadelphia Cream Cheese (1 oz.): 0/0. 15. Tribe All Natural Hummus Sweet Roasted Red Peppers (2 Tbsp.): 0/0. 16. Challenge Butter, whipped (1 Tbsp.): 0/0. 17. Organic Pastures Raw Butter (1 Tbsp.): 0/0.

**The Belly Fat Cure Seal of Approval has been awarded
to all Barlean's and Joseph's products above.**

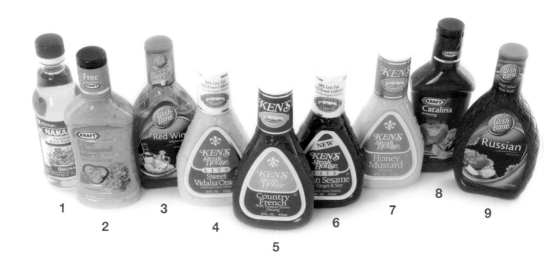

BELLY BAD

1. Mizkan Nakano Original Seasoned Rice Vinegar (2 Tbsp.): 5/1. 2. Kraft Free Thousand Island Fat Free Dressing (2 Tbsp.): 5/1. 3. Wish-Bone Red Wine Vinaigrette (2 Tbsp.): 8/1. 4. Ken's Steak House Lite Sweet Vidalia Onion Dressing (2 Tbsp.): 10/1. 5. Ken's Steak House Country French with Vermont Honey Dressing (2 Tbsp.): 9/1. 6. Ken's Steak House Lite Asian Sesame Dressing (2 Tbsp.): 7/1. 7. Ken's Steak House Honey Mustard Dressing (2 Tbsp.): 6/1. 8. Kraft Catalina Dressing (2 Tbsp.): 7/1. 9. Wish-Bone Russian Dressing (2 Tbsp.): 6/1.

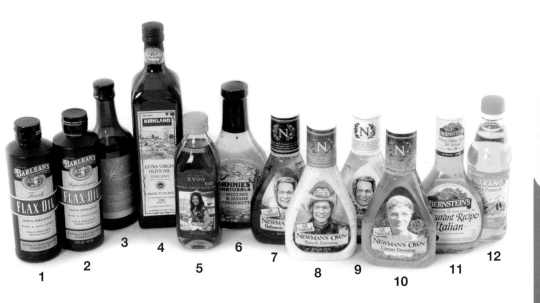

BELLY GOOD

1. Barlean's Fresh Flax Oil (1 Tbsp.): 0/0. 2. Barlean's Highest Lignan Flax Oil (1 Tbsp.): 0/0. 3. Living Harvest Hemp Oil (2 Tbsp.): 0/0. 4. Kirkland Signature Extra Virgin Olive Oil (1 Tbsp.): 0/0. 5. Rachael Ray EVOO Extra Virgin Olive Oil (1 Tbsp.): 0/0. 6. Annie's Naturals Shiitake & Sesame Vinaigrette (2 Tbsp.): 1/0. 7. Newman's Own Balsamic Vinaigrette (2 Tbsp.): 1/0. 8. Newman's Own Ranch Dressing (2 Tbsp.): 1/0. 9. Newman's Own Olive Oil & Vinegar Dressing (2 Tbsp.): 1/0. 10. Newman's Own Caesar Dressing (2 Tbsp.): 1/0. 11. Bernstein's Restaurant Recipe Italian Dressing (2 Tbsp.): 0/0. 12. Mizkan Nakano Natural Rice Vinegar (1 Tbsp.): 0/0.

**The Belly Fat Cure Seal of Approval has been awarded
to the Barlean's products above.**

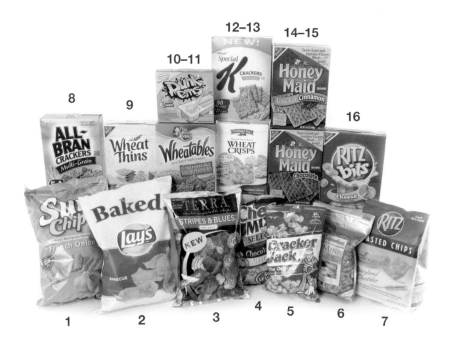

BELLY BAD

1. Sun Chips French Onion (1 oz.): 3/1. 2. Baked! Lay's Barbecue (1 oz.): 3/2. 3. Terra Stripes & Blues Sea Salt Chips (1 oz.): 5/1. 4. General Mills Chocolate Turtle Chex Mix Select (½ cup): 8/1. 5. Cracker Jack (½ cup): 15/2. 6. Inspirations Minis Sweet Maui Onion Pretzels (12 pretzels): 7/1. 7. Nabisco Toasted Chips Ritz Dairyland Cheddar (1 oz.): 3/1. 8. Kellogg's All-Bran Crackers Multi-Grain (18 crackers): 4/1. 9. Nabisco Wheat Thins Parmesan Basil (15 crackers): 4/2. 10. Kraft Handi-Snacks Dunk 'Ems Totally Cheesy (1 package): 4/1. 11. Keebler Wheatables Golden Wheat Reduced Fat (19 crackers): 5/2. 12. Kellogg's Special K Crackers Multi-Grain (24 crackers): 6/2. 13. Pepperidge Farm Baked Naturals Wheat Crisps Toasted Wheat (17 crackers): 5/2. 14. Nabisco Honey Maid Grahams Low Fat Cinnamon (2 full crackers): 10/2. 15. Nabisco Honey Maid Grahams Chocolate (2 full crackers): 9/2. 16. Nabisco Ritz Bits Cheese (13 bits): 4/1.

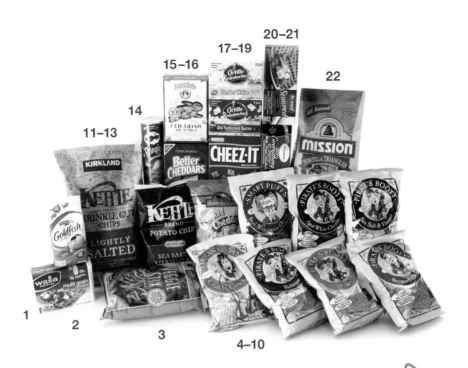

Labels on image: 20–21, 17–19, 15–16, 22, 14, 11–13, 1, 2, 3, 4–10

BELLY GOOD

1. Wasa Multi Grain Crispbread (1 slice): 0/1. 2. Pepperidge Farm Goldfish Crackers (55 pieces): 0/1. 3. Good Health Natural Products Veggie Stix (1 oz.): 0/1. 4. Original Tings (1 oz.): 0/1. 5. Pirate's Booty Barbeque Snack (1 oz.): 0/2. 6. Pirate's Booty Veggie Snack (1 oz.): 0/1. 7. Pirate's Booty Bermuda Onion Snack (1 oz.): 0/1. 8. Smart Puffs (1 oz.): 1/1. 9. Pirate's Booty Aged White Cheddar Snack (1 oz.): 0/1. 10. Pirate's Booty Sea Salt & Vinegar Snack (1 oz.): 0/1. 11. Kirkland Signature Kettle Brand Krinkle Cut Chips Lightly Salted (1 oz.): 0/1. 12. Kettle Brand Chips Sea Salt & Vinegar (1 oz.): 0/1. 13. Garden of Eatin' Baked Cheddar Puffs (1 oz.): 1/1. 14. Pringles Original Chips (1 oz.): 0/1. 15. Annie's Homegrown Cheddar Bunnies (50 crackers): 0/1. 16. Nabisco Better Cheddars (22 crackers): 0/1. 17. Orville Redenbacher's Tender White Popcorn (2 Tbsp. unpopped): 0/1. 18. Orville Redenbacher's Old Fashioned Butter Popcorn (2 Tbsp. unpopped): 0/1. 19. Sunshine Cheez-It Crackers (27 crackers): 0/1. 20. RyKrisp Seasoned Crackers (2 crackers): 0/1. 21. Milton's Everything Multi-Grain Crackers (2 crackers): 1/1. 22. Mission Restaurant Style Tortilla Triangles (10 chips): 0/1.

**The Belly Fat Cure Seal of Approval has been awarded
to all Pirate's Booty products above, including Original Tings and Smart Puffs.**

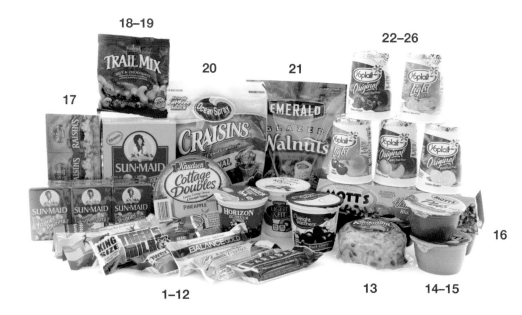

BELLY BAD

1. Clif Bar Chocolate Chip Peanut Crunch (1 bar): 21/3. 2. Luna Bar Nutz Over Chocolate (1 bar): 12/2. 3. Tiger's Milk Peanut Butter King Size Bar (1 bar): 20/2. 4. PowerBar Harvest Double Chocolate Crisp Bar (1 bar): 21/3. 5. Balance Gold Caramel Nut Blast Bar (1 bar): 14/2. 6. Fruitified ZonePerfect Strawberry Yogurt Bar (1 bar): 15/2. 7. Lärabar Cherry Pie (1 bar): 21/2. 8. Snack Size Sun-Maid Vanilla Yogurt Raisins (1 box): 18/1. 9. Knudsen Cottage Doubles Pineapple (1 container): 14/1. 10. Horizon Organic Blueberry Lowfat Blended Yogurt (1 container): 26/2. 11. Dannon Light & Fit Strawberry Kiwi Yogurt (1 container): 11/1. 12. Weight Watchers Black Cherry Yogurt (1 container): 12/1. 13. Kaukauna Sharp Cheddar Cheese Ball (2 Tbsp.): 4/0. 14. Mott's Classic Apple Sauce Cinnamon (4 oz.): 23/2. 15. Mott's Plus Fiber Sauce Cranberry Raspberry (4 oz.): 11/1. 16. Mott's Healthy Harvest Sauce Blueberry Delight (4 oz.): 11/1. 17. Del Monte Raisins (1 box): 29/2. 18. Planters Nut & Chocolate Trail Mix (1 package): 12/1. 19. Sun-Maid Golden Raisins (¼ cup): 29/2. 20. Ocean Spray Craisins (⅓ cup): 26/2. 21. Emerald Original Glazed Walnuts (1 oz.): 9/1. 22. Yoplait Light Very Cherry (1 container): 14/1. 23. Yoplait Original Harvest Peach (1 container): 27/2. 24. Yoplait Original Lemon Burst (1 container): 31/2. 25. Yoplait Original Mixed Berry (1 container): 27/2. 26. Yoplait Light Apricot Mango (1 container): 14/1. Contains aspartame.

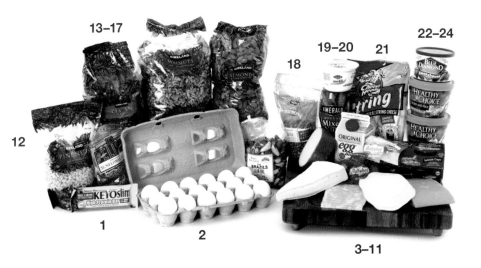

BELLY GOOD

1. Nature's Plus KETOslim High Protein Bar (1 bar): 2/2. 2. Egg (1 large): 0/0. 3. Safeway Select Smoked Gouda Cheese (1 oz.): 0/0. 4. Primo Taglio French Brie Cheese (1 oz.): 0/0. 5. Sargento Deli Style Sliced Colby-Jack Cheese (1 slice): 0/0. 6. The Laughing Cow Mini Babybel Original Semisoft Cheese (1 piece): 0/0. 7. Lucerne Provolone Cheese (1 slice): 0/0. 8. Lucerne Medium Cheddar Cheese (1 slice): 0/0. 9. Egg Beaters Original (¼ cup): 0/0. 10. Chicken of the Sea Salmon Cups (1 cup): 0/0. 11. Chicken of the Sea Chunk White Tuna Cups (1 cup): 0/0. 12. Kirkland Signature Pine Nuts (1 oz.): 1/0. 13. It's Delish! Sunflower Seeds (1 oz.): 1/1. 14. Kirkland Signature Pecan Halves (1 oz.): 1/0. 15. Kirkland Signature Walnuts (1 oz.): 1/0. 16. Kirkland Signature Almonds (1 oz.): 1/1. 17. Bates Nut Farm Raw Brazils (1 oz.): 1/0. 18. Emerald Harmony Roasted Soynuts (¼ cup): 0/1. 19. FAGE Total Yogurt (5.3 oz.): 5/1. 20. Emerald Deluxe Mixed Nuts (1 oz.): 1/1. 21. Frigo Cheese Heads StringCheese (1 oz.): 0/0. 22. Blue Diamond Smokehouse Almonds (1 oz.): 1/0. 23. Healthy Choice Chicken with Rice Soup (½ can): 0/1. 24. Healthy Choice Old Fashioned Chicken Noodle Soup (½ can): 0/1.

**The Belly Fat Cure Seal of Approval has been awarded
to all egg products above.**

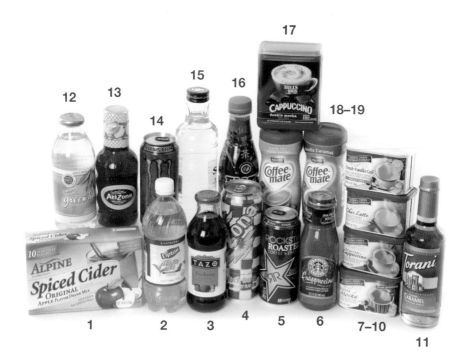

BELLY BAD

1. Alpine Original Spiced Cider Mix (1 packet): 20/1. 2. Lipton White Tea with Raspberry (1 bottle): 40/2. 3. Tazo Tazoberry Juiced Tea (1 bottle): 44/3. 4. Arizona Iced Tea with Raspberry Flavor (1 can): 66/4. 5. Rockstar Roasted Coffee & Energy Drink Mocha (1 can): 34/2. 6. Starbucks Dark Chocolate Mocha Frappuccino Coffee Drink (1 bottle): 48/3. 7. General Foods International Sugar Free French Vanilla Café (1⅓ Tbsp.): 0/0. Contains aspartame. 8. General Foods International Chai Latte (1⅓ Tbsp.): 10/1. 9. General Foods International Italian Cappuccino (1⅓ Tbsp.): 8/1. 10. General Foods International Suisse Mocha (1⅓ Tbsp.): 8/1. 11. Torani Caramel Syrup (2 Tbsp.): 19/1. 12. Snapple Green Tea (1 bottle): 30/2. 13. Arizona Lemon Iced Tea (1 bottle): 48/3. 14. Java Monster Russian (1 can): 34/2. 15. SoBe Green Tea (1 bottle): 61/4. 16. Fuze Black & Green Tea (1 bottle): 30/2. 17. Hills Bros. Double Mocha Cappuccino (3 Tbsp.): 15/0. 18. Coffee-mate Sugar Free French Vanilla Powder (1 Tbsp.): 0/0. Contains sucralose. 19. Coffee-mate Vanilla Caramel Powder (4 tsp.): 7/1.

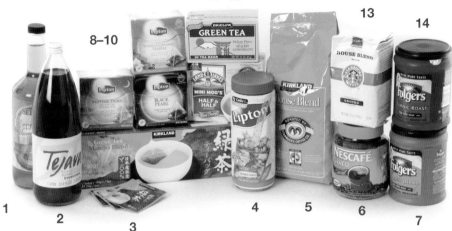

BELLY GOOD

1. Seelect Teas' Organic Caramel Syrup (2 oz.): 0/0. 2. Tejava Premium Iced Tea (8 oz.): 0/0. 3. Kirkland Signature Green Tea Matcha Blend (1 bag): 0/0. 4. Lipton Unsweetened Decaffeinated Lemon Iced Tea Mix (2 Tbsp.): 0/0. 5. Kirkland Signature House Blend Roasted by Starbucks Coffee Co. (2 Tbsp.): 0/0. 6. Nestlé Nescafé Clasico Decaf (2 Tbsp.): 0/0. 7. Folgers Classic Decaf Ground Coffee (2 Tbsp.): 0/0. 8. Lipton Bedtime Story Herbal Tea (1 bag): 0/0. 9. Lipton Black Pearl Tea (1 bag): 0/0. 10. Lipton Vanilla Caramel Truffle Tea (1 bag): 0/0. 11. Bigelow Green Tea (1 bag): 0/0. 12. Land O' Lakes Mini Moo's Half & Half (1 creamer): 0/0. 13. Starbucks House Blend Coffee (2 Tbsp.): 0/0. 14. Folgers Classic Roast Ground Coffee (2 Tbsp.): 0/0.

The Belly Fat Cure Seal of Approval has been awarded to all Kirkland products above.

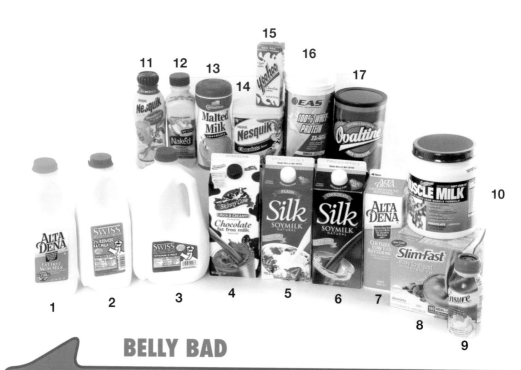

BELLY BAD

1. Alta Dena Fat Free Skim Milk (1 cup): 13/1. 2. Swiss Dairy 2% Reduced Fat Milk (1 cup): 14/1. 3. Swiss Dairy Vitamin D Whole Milk (1 cup): 12/1. 4. The Skinny Cow Fat Free Chocolate Milk (1 cup): 25/2. 5. Silk Plain Soymilk (1 cup): 6/1. 6. Silk Chocolate Soymilk (1 cup): 19/2. 7. Alta Dena Cultured Low Fat Buttermilk (1 cup): 13/1. 8. Slim-Fast Easy to Digest Chocolate Shake (1 can): 21/2. 9. Ensure Homemade Vanilla Shake (1 bottle): 23/2. 10. CytoSport Muscle Milk Chocolate Powder (1 scoop): 2/1. Contains sucralose. 11. Nestlé Nesquik Strawberry Milk (1 cup): 31/2. 12. Naked Juice Protein Zone Smoothie (1 bottle): 56/4. 13. Nestlé Carnation Chocolate Malted Milk (3 Tbsp.): 14/1. 14. Nestlé Nesquik Chocolate Powder (2 Tbsp.): 13/1. 15. Yoo-hoo Chocolate Drink (6.5 oz.): 18/2. 16. EAS 100% Whey Protein Vanilla (1 scoop): 1/0. Contains sucralose. 17. Ovaltine Rich Chocolate Mix (4 Tbsp.): 18/1.

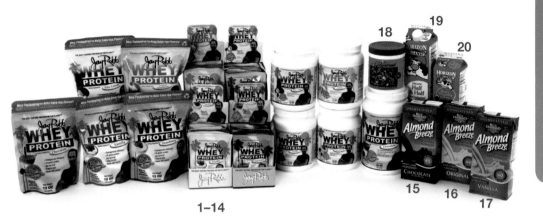

1–14

18 19 20

15 16 17

BELLY GOOD

1–14. Jay Robb Whey Protein in Chocolate, Vanilla, Tropical Dreamsicle, Strawberry, or Piña Colada (30 grams): 0/0. 15. Almond Breeze Chocolate Unsweetened Almond Milk (8 oz.): 0/0. 16. Almond Breeze Original Unsweetened Almond Milk (8 oz.): 0/0. 17. Almond Breeze Vanilla Unsweetened Almond Milk (8 oz.): 0/0. 18. Amazing Grass Kidz SuperFood Outrageous Chocolate Flavor (1 scoop): 1/0. 19. Horizon Organic Half & Half (2 Tbsp.): 1/0. 20. Horizon Organic Heavy Whipping Cream (1 Tbsp.): 0/0.

**The Belly Fat Cure Seal of Approval has been awarded
to all Jay Robb and Amazing Grass products above.**

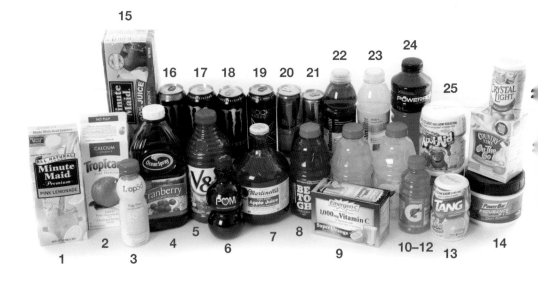

BELLY BAD

1. Minute Maid Pink Lemonade (8 oz.): 29/2. 2. Tropicana Pure Premium Orange Juice (8 oz.): 22/2. 3. Tropicana Trop50 (12 oz.): 15/1. 4. Ocean Spray Cranberry Juice Cocktail (8 oz.): 30/2. 5. V8 100% Vegetable Juice (8 oz.): 8/1. 6. POM Wonderful 100% Pomegranate Juice (8 oz.): 32/2. 7. Martinelli's Apple Juice (8 oz.): 31/2. 8. Gatorade Fruit Punch (8 oz.): 14/1. 9. Emergen-C Super Orange (1 packet): 5/1. 10. Gatorade Frost Glacier Freeze (8 oz.): 14/1. 11. Gatorade Lemon-Lime (8 oz.): 14/1. 12. Gatorade Orange (12 oz.): 21/2. 13. Tang Orange Powder (⅛ cap): 9/1. 14. PowerBar Endurance Fruit Punch Sports Drink (1 scoop): 9/1. 15. Minute Maid Fruit Punch (1 box): 21/2. 16. Monster Mixxd (1 can): 54/3. 17. Lo-Carb Monster Energy (1 can): 6/1. Contains sucralose. 18. Monster Energy (1 can): 54/3. 19. Original Rockstar Energy Drink (1 can): 62/4. 20. Red Bull Energy Drink (12 oz.): 39/2. 21. Red Bull Sugarfree Energy Drink (8.4 oz.): 0/0. Contains aspartame. 22. Glacéau Vitaminwater XXX (Acai-Blueberry-Pomegranate) (1 bottle): 33/2. 23. Glacéau Vitaminwater Multi-V (Lemonade) (1 bottle): 33/2. 24. Powerade Fruit Punch (8 oz.): 14/1. 25. Kool-Aid Tropical Punch (⅛ cap): 16/1. 26. Country Time On the Go Lemonade (1 packet): 18/1. 27. Crystal Light Pink Lemonade (⅛ tub): 0/0. Contains aspartame.

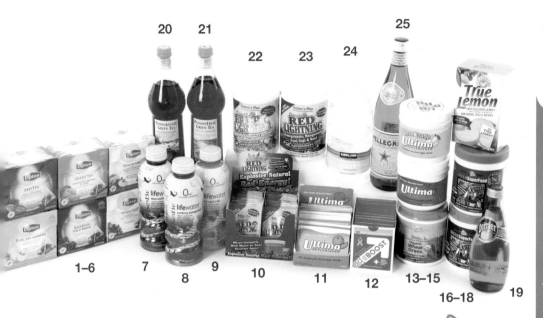

BELLY GOOD

1. Lipton Tuscan Lemon Tea (1 bag): 0/0. 2. Lipton Bavarian Wild Berry Tea (1 bag): 0/0. 3. Lipton White Tea with Blueberry & Pomegranate Flavor (1 bag): 0/0. 4. Lipton Red Tea with Harvest Strawberry & Passionfruit Flavor (1 bag): 0/0. 5. Lipton Green Tea with Mandarin Orange Flavor (1 bag): 0/0. 6. Lipton White Tea with Island Mango & Peach Flavors (1 bag): 0/0. 7. SoBe Black and Blue Berry Lifewater (1 bottle): 0/1. 8. SoBe Yumberry Pomegranate Lifewater (1 bottle): 0/1. 9. SoBe Fuji Apple Pear Lifewater (1 bottle): 0/1. 10. Nature's Plus Source of Life Red Lightning (2 tsp.): 0/0. 11. Ultima Replenisher Orange (1 packet): 0/0. 12. EBoost Pink Lemonade (1 packet): 0/0. 13. Amazing Grass Organic Wheat Grass Powder (1 Tbsp.): 0/0. 14. Ultima Replenisher Wild Raspberry (1 packet): 0/0. 15. Ultima Replenisher Lemonade (1 packet): 0/0. 16. Amazing Grass Green SuperFood Chocolate Drink Powder (1 scoop): 0/0. 17. Amazing Grass Green SuperFood Berry Flavor Drink Powder (1 scoop): 0/0. 18. True Lemon (1 packet): 0/0. 19. Perrier Lemon (1 bottle): 0/0. 20. The Republic of Tea Pomegranate Green Tea Iced Tea (1 bottle): 0/0. 21. The Republic of Tea PassionFruit Green Tea Iced Tea (1 bottle): 0/0. 22. Nature's Plus Source of Life Bright Lightning (2 tsp.): 0/0. 23. Nature's Plus Source of Life Red Lightning (2 tsp.): 0/0. 24. Kirkland Signature Water (1 bottle): 0/0. 25. S.Pellegrino Sparkling Natural Mineral Water (8 oz.): 0/0.

**The Belly Fat Cure Seal of Approval has been awarded
to all Amazing Grass products above.**

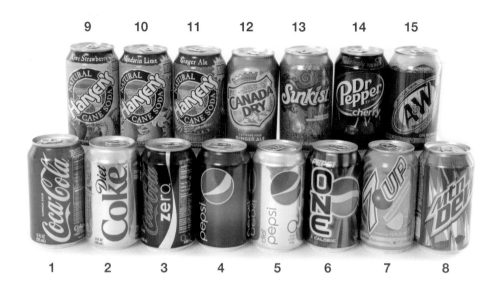

BELLY BAD

1. Coca-Cola (1 can): 41/3. 2. Diet Coke (1 can): 0/0. Contains aspartame. 3. Coca-Cola Zero (1 can): 0/0. Contains aspartame. 4. Pepsi (1 can): 41/3. 5. Diet Pepsi (1 can): 0/0. Contains aspartame. 6. Pepsi One (1 can): 0/0. Contains sucralose. 7. 7UP (1 can): 38/2. 8. Mountain Dew (1 can): 46/3. 9. Hansen's Kiwi Strawberry Natural Cane Soda (1 can): 37/2. 10. Hansen's Mandarin Lime Natural Cane Soda (1 can): 39/2. 11. Hansen's Ginger Ale Natural Cane Soda (1 can): 44/3. 12. Canada Dry Ginger Ale (1 can): 35/2. 13. Sunkist Orange Soda (1 can): 50/3. 14. Dr Pepper Cherry (1 can): 41/3. 15. A&W Root Beer (1 can): 45/3.

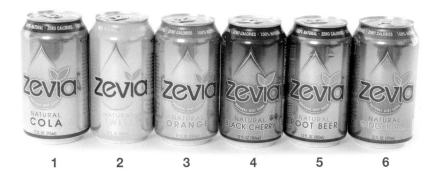

1   2   3   4   5   6

BELLY GOOD

1. Zevia Natural Cola (1 can): 0/1. 2. Zevia Natural Twist (1 can): 0/1. 3. Zevia Natural Orange (1 can): 0/1. 4. Zevia Natural Black Cherry (1 can): 0/1. 5. Zevia Natural Root Beer (1 can): 0/1. 6. Zevia Natural Ginger Ale (1 can): 0/1.

**The Belly Fat Cure Seal of Approval has been awarded
to all Zevia products above.**

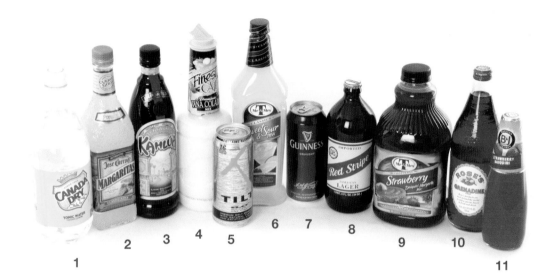

BELLY BAD

1. Canada Dry Tonic Water (8 oz.): 23/1. 2. Jose Cuervo Classic Lime Margaritas (4 oz.): 24/2. 3. Kahlúa (1 oz.): 15/1. 4. Finest Call Piña Colada Mix (4 oz.): 52/3. 5. Anheuser-Busch Tilt Green (12 oz.): 7/3. 6. Mr & Mrs T Sweet & Sour Mix (4 oz.): 22/2. 7. Guinness (12 oz.): 6/1. 8. Red Stripe Lager (12 oz.): 14/1. 9. Mr & Mrs T Strawberry Daiquiri-Margarita Mix (4 oz.): 44/3. 10. Rose's Grenadine (2 Tbsp.): 20/2. 11. Bartles & Jaymes Strawberry Daiquiri (12 oz.): 33/2.

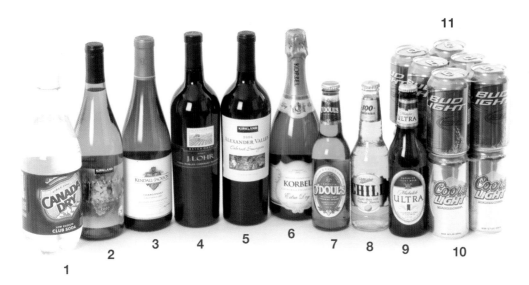

BELLY GOOD

1. Canada Dry Club Soda (8 oz.): 0/0. 2. Kirkland Signature Chardonnay (5 oz.): 0/0. 3. Kendall-Jackson Chardonnay (5 oz.): 0/0. 4. J. Lohr Cabernet Sauvignon (5 oz.): 0/1. 5. Kirkland Signature Cabernet Sauvignon (5 oz.): 0/1. 6. Korbel Extra Dry California Champagne (4 oz.): 0/0. 7. O'Doul's Non-Alcoholic Brew (12 oz.): 0/1. 8. Miller Chill (12 oz.): 0/0. 9. Michelob Ultra (12 oz.): 0/0. 10. Coors Light (12 oz.): 0/1. 11. Bud Light (12 oz.): 0/1.

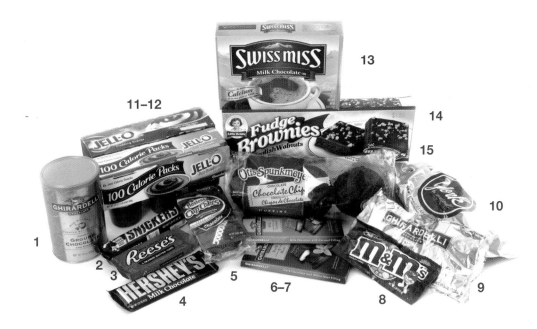

BELLY BAD

1. Ghirardelli Sweet Ground Chocolate and Cocoa (¼ cup): 31/2. 2. King Size Snickers (1 bar): 23/2. 3. Reese's Peanut Butter Cups (1 package): 20/2. 4. Hershey's Milk Chocolate (1 bar): 24/2. 5. Hostess Cup Cakes (2 cakes): 44/4. 6. Ghirardelli Dark Chocolate with Mint Filling Bar (3 pieces): 20/2. 7. Ghirardelli Milk Chocolate with Caramel Filling Bar (3 pieces): 20/2. 8. Milk Chocolate M&M's (1 pack): 31/2. 9. Ghirardelli Milk Chocolate Chips (16 chips): 10/1. 10. York Dark Chocolate Covered Peppermint Patties (3 patties): 26/2. 11. Jell-O Chocolate Vanilla Swirl Pudding Snacks (1 snack): 19/2. 12. Jell-O Fat Free Chocolate Pudding Snacks (1 snack): 17/2. 13. Swiss Miss Milk Chocolate Hot Cocoa (1 packet): 16/2. 14. Little Debbie Fudge Brownies (1 brownie): 21/2. 15. Otis Spunkmeyer Chocolate Chocolate Chip Muffins (1 muffin): 32/3.

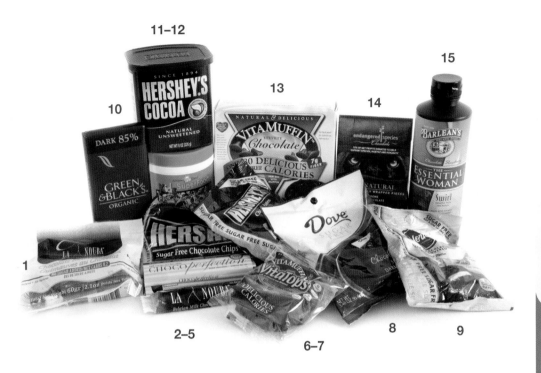

11–12

10

13

14

15

1

2–5

6–7

8

9

BELLY GOOD

1. La Nouba Chocolate Covered Marshmallows (1 piece): 0/1. 2. La Nouba Raspberry Belgian Milk Chocolate Bar (1 bar): 0/2. 3. LowCarb Specialties, Inc. ChocoPerfection Milk Chocolate Bar (1 bar): 0/1. 4. LowCarb Specialties, Inc. ChocoPerfection Dark Chocolate Bar (1 bar): 0/1. 5. Hershey's Sugar Free Chocolate Chips (1 Tbsp.): 0/1. 6. Vitalicious Sugar Free Velvety Chocolate VitaTop (1 top): 0/2. 7. Hershey's Sugar Free Chocolates (5 pieces): 0/2. 8. Dove Sugar Free Chocolate Crème Dark Chocolates (5 pieces): 0/2. 9. York Sugar Free Peppermint Patties (3 pieces): 0/2. 10. Green & Black's Organic Dark 85% Chocolate (12 pieces): 5/1. 11. Hershey's Natural Unsweetened Cocoa (1 Tbsp.): 0/0. 12. Amazing Grass Kidz SuperFood Outrageous Chocolate Flavor (1 scoop): 0/0. 13. Vitalicious Velvety Chocolate VitaMuffins (1 muffin): 0/2. 14. Endangered Species Chocolate All Natural Extreme Dark Chocolate (4 pieces): 5/1. 15. Barlean's Chocolate Raspberry Omega Swirl (1 Tbsp.): 0/0.

**The Belly Fat Cure Seal of Approval has been awarded
to all Barlean's and Sugar Free VitaMuffin products above.**

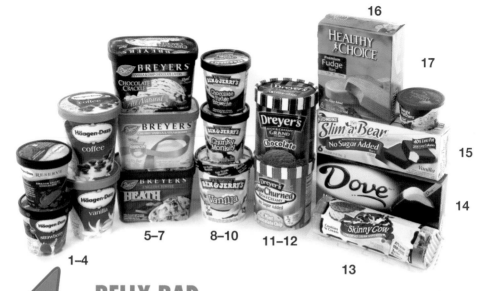

BELLY BAD

1. Häagen-Dazs Strawberry (½ cup): 20/2. 2. Häagen-Dazs Reserve Amazon Valley Chocolate (½ cup): 21/2. 3. Häagen-Dazs Vanilla (½ cup): 19/1. 4. Häagen-Dazs Coffee (½ cup): 19/2. 5. Breyers Heath English Toffee (½ cup): 20/2. 6. Breyers Double Churn Light Creamy Vanilla & Strawberry (½ cup): 13/1. 7. Breyers All Natural Chocolate Crackle (½ cup): 15/1. 8. Ben & Jerry's Vanilla (½ cup): 19/2. 9. Ben & Jerry's Chunky Monkey (¼ cup): 27/2. 10. Ben & Jerry's Chocolate Fudge Brownie (½ cup): 25/2. 11. Dreyer's Slow Churned No Sugar Added Mint Chocolate Chip (½ cup): 3/1. Contains sucralose. 12. Dreyer's Grand Chocolate (½ cup): 15/1. 13. The Skinny Cow Cookies 'N Cream Low Fat Ice Cream Sandwiches (1 sandwich): 15/2. 14. Dove Milk Chocolate with Vanilla Ice Cream Bar (1 bar): 22/2. 15. Klondike Slim-a-Bear No Sugar Added (1 sandwich): 7/2. Contains aspartame. 16. Healthy Choice Premium Fudge Bars (1 bar): 4/1. Contains Aspartame. 17. Weight Watchers Cookies & Cream Cup (1 cup): 21/2.

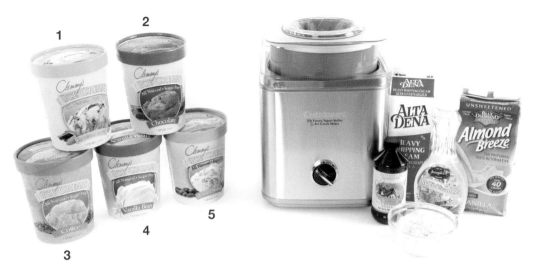

BELLY GOOD

1. Clemmy's Chocolate Mint Swirl (½ cup): 0/1. 2. Clemmy's Chocolate (½ cup): 0/1. 3. Clemmy's Coffee (½ cup): 0/1. 4. Clemmy's Vanilla Bean (½ cup): 0/1. 5. Clemmy's Toasted Almond (½ cup): 0/1.

In case you can't find Clemmy's at your local store, you can try my simple recipe for homemade ice cream (you'll need an ice-cream maker):

FOUR-INGREDIENT HOMEMADE VANILLA ICE CREAM*
Serves: 14 (½ cup serving); S/C Value = 0/0

INGREDIENTS
1½ cups unsweetened vanilla almond milk
1⅛ cups maltitol sweetener syrup*
3 cups heavy whipping cream
1½ Tbsp. pure vanilla extract

PREPARATION
1. In a medium mixing bowl, mix together all listed ingredients.

2. Turn the ice-cream maker on; pour the mixture into the freezer bowl and let mix until thickened, about 20–25 minutes. The ice cream will be ready to eat with a soft and creamy texture. If a firmer consistency is desired, transfer the ice cream to an airtight container and freeze for about 2 hours.

* Note: This recipe is for a 2-quart ice-cream maker. We also used Joseph's brand of maltitol sweetener, which is available at: josephslitecookies.com.

**The Belly Fat Cure Seal of Approval has been awarded
to all Clemmy's products above.**

BELLY BAD

1. Nabisco SnackWell's Creme Sandwich Cookies (1 package): 18/2. 2. Nabisco Nutter Butter (1 package): 15/2. 3. Nabisco Teddy Grahams Cinnamon (24 pieces): 8/2. 4. Starburst Tropical Fruit Chews (1 package): 34/3. 5. Mentos Fruit Chewy Mints (1 piece): 2/0. 6. Skittles Original Fruit (1 bag): 47/3. 7. Sour Patch Watermelon (1 package): 36/3. 8. Hot Tamales (1 package): 39/3. 9. Starburst GummiBursts (1 bag): 23/2. 10. Jelly Belly Jelly Beans (35 pieces): 28/2. 11. CVS Peppermint Candy (3 pieces): 10/1. 12. Twizzlers Strawberry Twists (6 pieces): 18/2. 13–18. Trident Sugarless Gum (1 piece): 0/0. Contains aspartame. 19. Hostess Raspberry Zingers (3 cakes): 51/4. 20. Hostess Twinkies (2 cakes): 35/3. 21. Nabisco Reduced Fat Nilla Wafers (8 wafers): 12/2. 22. Pepperidge Farm Milano Cookies (3 cookies): 13/2. 23. Kellogg's Pop-Tarts Frosted Strawberry (1 pastry): 20/2. 24. Keebler Soft Batch Chocolate Chip Cookies (1 package): 23/3. 25. Nabisco Oreo Cakesters (1 package): 33/3. 26. Nabisco Fig Newtons (2 cookies): 12/2. 27. Nabisco Chips Ahoy! (3 cookies): 10/2. 28. Kellogg's Rice Krispies Treats (1 bar): 7/1. 29. Nabisco Chips Ahoy! Reduced Fat (3 cookies): 11/2. 30. Nabisco Oreo (3 cookies): 14/2. 31. Hershey's Chocolate Syrup (2 Tbsp.): 20/2. 32. Hershey's Strawberry Syrup (2 Tbsp.): 24/2. 33. Smucker's Caramel Flavored Sundae Syrup (2 Tbsp.): 20/2. 34. Kraft Cool Whip (2 Tbsp.): 1/0. 35. Wrigley's Juicy Fruit (1 stick): 2/0. 36. Wrigley's Doublemint (1 stick): 2/0. 37. Bubble Yum (1 piece): 5/1. 38–39. Wrigley's Orbit Gum (1 stick): 0/0. Contains aspartame. 40. Wrigley's Big Red (1 stick): 2/0. Contains aspartame. 41. Jell-O Sugar-Free Vanilla Pudding Snacks (1 snack): 0/1. Contains sucralose. 42. Jell-O Strawberry/Orange Gelatin Snacks (1 snack): 17/1.

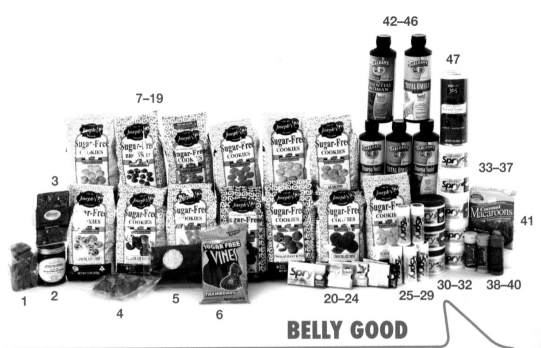

BELLY GOOD

1. Judy's Candy Company Sugar Free Vanilla Caramels (1 piece): 0/1. 2. Perfectly Sweet Sugar Free Pecan Praline Sauce (2 Tbsp.): 0/1. 3. Judy's Candy Company Sugar Free Peanut Brittle (¾ cup): 0/2. 4. Perfectly Sweet Sugar Free Cinna Cubs (9 pieces): 0/2. 5. Perfectly Sweet Sugar Free Black Licorice Twist Stix (7 pieces): 0/2. 6. Red Vines Sugar Free Vines Strawberry (7 twists): 0/2. 7–19. Joseph's Sugar-Free Cookies (4 cookies): 0/1. 20–24. Xlear, Inc. Spry Sugar Free Gum (1 piece): 0/0. 25–29. Xlear, Inc. Spry Sugar Free Gum (1 piece): 0/0. 30–32. Xlear, Inc. Spry Sugar Free Mints (1 piece): 0/0. 33–37. Xlear, Inc. Spry Sugar Free Gum (1 piece): 0/0. 38–40. Xlear, Inc. SparX Candy (1 piece): 0/0. 41. Jennies Unsweetened Coconut Macaroons (2 cookies): 1/1. 42. Barlean's Lemon Zest Omega Swirl (2 tsp.): 0/0. 43. Barlean's Pomegranate Blueberry Total Omega Vegan Swirl (1 Tbsp.): 0/1. 44. Barlean's Strawberry Banana Omega Swirl (1 Tbsp.): 0/1. 45. Barlean's Chocolate Raspberry Omega Swirl (1 Tbsp.): 0/1. 46. Barlean's Orange Cream Omega Swirl (1 Tbsp.): 0/1. 47. 365 Everyday Value Real Dairy Nonfat Whipped Topping (2 Tbsp.): 0/0.

**The Belly Fat Cure Seal of Approval has been awarded
to all Barlean's, Joseph's, Spry, and Xlear, Inc., products above.**

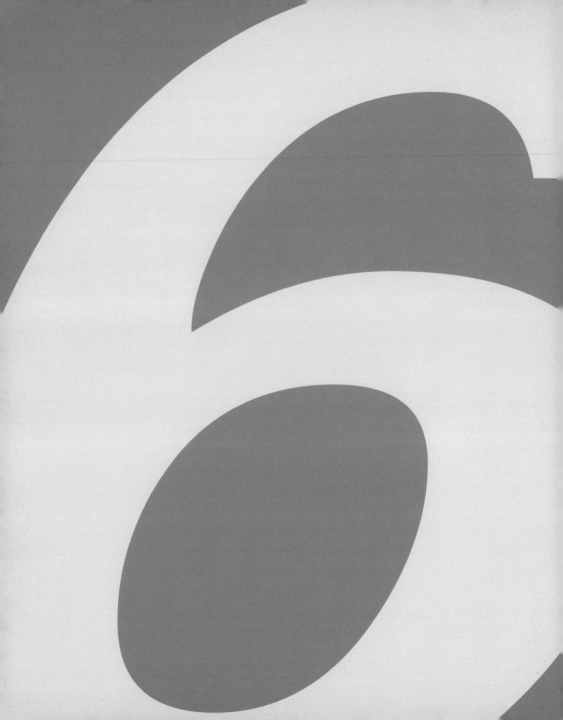

6

Carb Swap
Food List

Many of my clients have told me that the food list in this chapter is the most valuable tool for success on the Belly Fat Cure. With more than 800 items, this list will allow you to scan quickly and find the S/C Value of your favorite types of food, including those items used in our Belly Good meals. For example, a 1-oz. serving of chicken breast deli lunch meat has an S/C Value of 1/0.

Did you find a great product that we should add to our list? If so, please visit us at **TheBellyFatCure.com**.

FOOD LIST

FOOD ITEM	SERVING	S/C VALUE	FOOD ITEM	SERVING	S/C VALUE
1. POULTRY			Sausage, beef, precooked	1 oz.	0/0
Chicken breast, lunch meat, deli	1 oz.	1/0	Short ribs, lean, with bone, braised	1 rib	0/0
Chicken breast, premium chunk,	2 oz.	0/0	Steak, sirloin, strip, ⅛ trim, broiled	3 oz.	0/0
Kirkland Signature			Steak, top sirloin, lean broiled	3 oz.	0/0
Chicken liver, pâté	1 oz.	0/0	T-bone, lean, broiled	3 oz.	0/0
Chicken, breast, no skin, no sauces	3 oz.	0/0	Tenderloin, boneless, roasted	3 oz.	0/0
Chicken, dark meat, no skin, no sauces	3 oz.	0/0	Top round, steak, lean, braised	3 oz.	0/0
Chicken, drumstick, no skin, no sauces	1	0/0	Tri-tip roast, lean, roasted, Santa Maria style	3 oz.	0/0
Chicken, drumstick, with skin, no sauces	1	0/0			
Chicken, frozen, grilled strips, Foster Farms	3 oz.	0/0	Lamb		
Chicken, rotisserie, no skin, Kirkland Signature	3 oz.	0/0	Ground, broiled	3 oz.	0/0
Chicken, thigh, with bone, no skin, no sauces	1	0/0	Kebab, lean, braised	3 oz.	0/0
Chicken, thigh, with bone, with skin, no sauces	1	0/0	Loin chop, lean, broiled	3 oz.	0/0
Turkey bacon, extra lean, Jennie-O	.5 oz	0/0			
Turkey bacon, Oscar Mayer Louis Rich	.5 oz	0/0	Pork		
Turkey burger patties, 85/15, Jennie-O	1	0/0	Bacon, medium, cooked, slice	2	0/0
Turkey burger patties, Foster Farms	1	0/0	Canadian bacon, grilled, slice	2	0/0
Turkey meatballs, Foster Farms	3	0/1	Capicola, slice	2	0/0
Turkey sausage, links, Jimmy Dean	1	0/0	Chop, center lean, with bone, braised	2.6 oz.	0/0
Turkey, dark meat, no skin, no sauces	3 oz.	0/0	Chop, stuffed	5.5 oz.	0/2
Turkey, dark meat, with skin	3 oz.	0/0	Ground, cooked	3 oz.	0/0
Turkey, ground, 85% lean	3 oz.	0/0	Ham, boneless, 11% fat	4 oz.	1/0
Turkey, light meat, no skin, no sauces	3 oz.	0/0	Ham, deli	1 oz.	0/0
Turkey, light meat, with skin	3 oz.	0/0	Ham, slice, The HoneyBaked Ham Company	3	6/1
			Hot dog	1	0/0
2. MEATS			Prosciutto, slice	2	0/0
Beef			Ribs, country style, lean braised, no sauce	3 oz.	0/0
Bottom round, all lean, cooked	3 oz.	0/0	Roast, center loin, lean roasted	3 oz.	0/0
Brisket flat, lean, braised	3 oz.	0/0	Salami, Italian pork	1 oz.	0/0
Chuck roast, lean, braised	3 oz.	0/0	Sausage, crumbles, hot 'n spicy, Johnsonville	½ cup	0/0
Corned beef, cooked	3 oz.	1/1	Sausage, links, cooked	2	0/0
Cotto salami, beef	1 oz.	0/0	Sausage, patty, original, Jimmy Dean	1	1/0
Eye round, lean, roasted	3 oz.	0/0	Tenderloin, roasted	3 oz.	0/0
Filet mignon, lean, broiled	4 oz.	0/0			
Flank steak, lean, braised	3 oz.	0/0	**3. FISH & SEAFOOD**		
Ground, extra lean	4 oz.	0/0	Anchovies, with oil, drained	3 oz.	0/0
Hot dog, beef	1	2/0	Bass, sea	3 oz.	0/0
Jerky, beef	.7 oz.	2/0	Bass, striped	3 oz.	0/0
Pastrami, beef, deli	1 oz.	0/0	Carp	3 oz.	0/0
Rib pot roast, lean, roasted	3 oz.	0/0	Catfish	3 oz.	0/0
Rib steak, lean, roasted	3 oz.	0/0	Cod	3 oz.	0/0
Roast beef, deli	1 oz.	1/0	Crab legs, Alaskan King	3.5 oz.	0/0
Salami, beef, lean, sliced	1 oz.	0/0	Crab, blue, canned	½ cup	0/0

FOOD ITEM	SERVING	S/C VALUE
Crab, Dungeness	3 oz.	0/0
Crab, imitation	3 oz.	0/1
Crab, snow, leg	3 oz.	0/0
Fish roe	1 Tbsp.	0/0
Flounder	3 oz.	0/0
Grouper	3 oz.	0/0
Haddock	3 oz.	0/0
Halibut, Atlantic	3 oz.	0/0
Herring, Atlantic	3 oz.	0/0
Lobster	3 oz.	0/0
Mackerel, Atlantic	3 oz.	0/0
Mahimahi	3 oz.	0/0
Monkfish	3 oz.	0/0
Orange roughy	3 oz.	0/0
Perch	3 oz.	0/0
Pollock	3 oz.	0/0
Rockfish	3 oz.	0/0
Salmon, Atlantic, wild	3 oz.	0/0
Salmon, Chinook, smoked lox	1 oz.	0/0
Salmon, pink, canned	3 oz.	0/0
Sardines	1 oz.	0/0
Scallops	3	0/0
Shark	3 oz.	0/0
Shrimp	3 oz.	0/0
Snapper	3 oz.	0/0
Sole	3 oz.	0/0
Squid (fried calamari)	4 oz.	0/1
Sturgeon	3 oz.	0/0
Swordfish	3 oz.	0/0
Tilapia	3 oz.	0/0
Trout, rainbow	3 oz.	0/0
Tuna, bluefin	3 oz.	0/0
Tuna, chunk light, canned, in oil	3 oz.	0/0
Tuna, chunk light, canned, in water	3 oz.	0/0
Tuna, hickory smoked, Tuna Creations, Starkist	3 oz.	0/0
Tuna, skipjack	3 oz.	0/0
Tuna, yellowfin	3 oz.	0/0

4. EGGS

FOOD ITEM	SERVING	S/C VALUE
Egg substitute, original, Egg Beaters	¼ cup	0/0
Egg, Egg Starts, Kirkland Signature	¼ cup	0/0
Egg, large	1	0/0
Egg, whites	1	0/0

5. MEATLESS "MEATS"

FOOD ITEM	SERVING	S/C VALUE
Bacon, meatless, slice	1	0/0
Breakfast link, soy	1	1/0
Breakfast patty, Morningstar Farms	1	1/0
Burger patty, all American flame grilled, Boca	1	1/1
Burger patty, cheeseburger, Boca	1	1/1
Burger patty, grillers prime, Morningstar Farms	1	0/1
Burger patty, spicy black bean, Morningstar Farms	1	2/1
Canadian bacon, soy, slice, Yves	1	0/0
Chik'n nuggets, Morningstar Farms	4	3/1
Chik'n patty, Boca	1	1/1
Chorizo, soy, soyrizo, El Burrito	1.9 oz.	2/1
Grillers Recipe Crumbles, Meal Starters, Morningstar Farms	1.9 oz.	1/0
Ground beef style, Gimme Lean, Lightlife	3 oz.	2/1
Veggie dogs, veggie protein links, Lightlife	1	1/0
Veggie sausage, Italian style, Morningstar Farms	1	2/1
Pepperoni, soy, sliced	1 oz.	0/0
Sausage-style recipe crumbles, Meal Starters, Morningstar Farms	⅔ cup	0/1
Sausage, ground sausage style, Gimme Lean, Lightlife	2 oz.	1/0
Tofu, firm, raw	2.9 oz.	1/0
Veggie cakes, ginger teriyaki, Morningstar Farms	1	2/1

6. DAIRY & DAIRY REPLACEMENTS

FOOD ITEM	SERVING	S/C VALUE
Almond milk, chocolate, unsweetened, Almond Breeze	8 oz.	0/0
Almond milk, original, unsweetened, Almond Breeze	8 oz.	0/0
Almond milk, vanilla, unsweetened, Almond Breeze	8 oz.	0/0
Brie	1 oz.	0/0
Butter, European style, Challenge Butter	1 Tbsp.	0/0
Butter, raw, Organic Pasture	1 Tbsp.	0/0
Butter, unsalted, whipped, Challenge Butter	1 Tbsp.	0/0
Cheese, American	1 oz.	0/0
Cheese, Blue	1 Tbsp.	0/0
Cheese, cheddar	1 oz.	0/0
Cheese, colby-Jack, Sargento	1 oz.	0/0
Cheese, cotija	1 oz.	0/0

FOOD ITEM	SERVING	S/C VALUE
Cheese, feta	¼ cup	2/0
Cheese, French brie, Primo Taglio	1 oz.	0/0
Cheese, goat, semisoft	1 oz.	1/0
Cheese, gouda	1 oz.	1/0
Cheese, grated, Parmesan	¼ cup	0/0
Cheese, grated, Romano	1 oz.	0/0
Cheese, Gruyère	1 oz.	0/0
Cheese, Jarlsberg, Sargento	1 oz.	0/0
Cheese, Monterey Jack, fat free	1 oz.	0/0
Cheese, mozzarella, part skim	1 oz.	0/0
Cheese, mozzarella, string	1 oz.	0/0
Cheese, mozzarella, string, Frigo Cheese Heads	1 oz.	0/0
Cheese, Muenster	1 oz.	0/0
Cheese, Neufchâtel	1 oz.	0/0
Cheese, original wedges, The Laughing Cow	1	1/0
Cheese, pepper Jack	1 oz.	0/0
Cheese, provolone	1 oz.	0/0
Cheese, ricotta	½ cup	0/0
Cheese, Roquefort	1 oz.	0/0
Cheese, semisoft, Babybel, The Laughing Cow	1	0/0
Cheese, smoked gouda, Safeway Select	1 oz.	0/0
Cheese, soy, American, Tofutti	2 oz.	0/0
Cheese, Swiss	1 oz.	0/0
Cheese spread, old English, Kraft	2 Tbsp.	0/0
Cool whip, light, Kraft	2 Tbsp.	1/0
Cottage cheese, 2% low fat	¼ cup	0/0
Cream cheese, fat free	2 Tbsp.	0/0
Cream cheese, Philadelphia, Kraft	1 oz.	0/0
Cream, heavy	¼ cup	0/0
Half & half, Horizon Organic	2 Tbsp.	1/0
Half & half, Mini Moo's, Land O' Lakes	1	0/0
Heavy whipping cream, Alta Dena	1 Tbsp.	0/0
Ice cream, chocolate mint swirl, Clemmy's	½ cup	0/1
Ice cream, chocolate, Clemmy's	½ cup	0/1
Ice cream, coffee, Clemmy's	½ cup	0/1
Ice cream, toasted almond, Clemmy's	½ cup	0/1
Ice cream, vanilla bean, Clemmy's	½ cup	0/1
Margarine, with salt	1 Tbsp.	0/0
Milk, 1%	1 cup	12/1
Milk, nonfat	1 cup	12/1
Milk, nonfat, dry	3 Tbsp.	12/1
Milk, whole	1 cup	13/1

FOOD ITEM	SERVING	S/C VALUE
Rice drink, original, Rice Dream	1 cup	10/2
Sour cream	1 Tbsp.	0/0
Sour cream, Horizon Organic	1 Tbsp.	1/0
Spread, cream cheese, whipped garlic 'n herb, Philadelphia, Kraft	2 Tbsp.	1/0
Yogurt, organic fat-free plain, Stonyfield Farm	6 oz.	12/1
Yogurt, plain, 5%, FAGE	5.3 oz.	5/1

7. LEGUMES

Baked beans	½ cup	12/2
Baked beans, organic vegetarian, Amy's	½ cup	9/2
Baked beans, original, Bush Brothers	½ cup	12/2
Black beans, canned, Progresso	½ cup	0/1
Black beans, cooked	½ cup	0/1
Black-eyed peas, cooked	½ cup	1/1
Broad beans (cava), cooked	½ cup	0/1
Butter beans (lima), cooked	½ cup	1/1
Cannellini beans, cooked	½ cup	2/1
Chickpeas/garbanzo beans, cooked	½ cup	4/2
Edamame (shelled soybeans), cooked	½ cup	1/1
Hummus	⅛ cup	0/1
Kidney beans, boiled	½ cup	0/1
Lentils, brown, boiled	½ cup	2/1
Navy beans, cooked	½ cup	0/1
Pinto beans, cooked	½ cup	0/2
Refried beans	½ cup	0/1
Split peas, cooked	½ cup	3/1
White beans, cooked	½ cup	1/1

8. BREADS, CRACKERS & TORTILLAS

Bagel, multigrain, Rudi's Organic Bakery	1	3/2
Bagel, plain, Rudi's Organic Bakery	1	3/2
Bagel, sprouted wheat, Alvarado Street Bakery	1	2/3
Bread, crumbs, panko, Ian's	2 Tbsp.	0/1
Bread, light brown rice loaf, Ener-G	1 pita	1/1
Bread, pita, 100% whole wheat, Mr. Pita, Sara Lee	1 pita	0/1
Bread, pita pocket, whole wheat, 6½"	1 pita	1/2
Bread, prophets pocket, Food for Life Ezekiel 4:9	1 pita	1/2
Bread, sprouted grain bread low sodium, Food for Life Ezekiel 4:9	1 slice	0/1
Bread, sprouted whole grain, Food for Life	1 slice	0/1

FOOD ITEM	SERVING	S/C VALUE
Ezekiel 4:9		
Bread, whole wheat, light, Oroweat	1 slice	2/1
Crackers, crispbread, multi grain, Wasa	1 slice	0/1
Crackers, matzo, whole wheat	1 oz.	1/1
Crackers, melba toast, plain	.75 oz.	0/1
Crackers, original, Ritz, Nabisco	.6 oz.	1/1
Crackers, saltine, Nabisco	.5 oz.	0/1
Crackers, Triscuit, Nabisco	1 oz.	0/1
Crackers, Wheat Thins, Nabisco	.6 oz.	2/1
English muffin, sprouted grain, Food for Life Ezekiel 4:9	½	0/1
English muffin, whole grain, Rudi's Organic Bakery	1	2/2
Flour tortillas, garden spinach & vegetables, Tumaro's	1	1/2
Flour tortillas, sun-dried tomato & basil, Tumaro's	1	1/2
Flour, organic soy flour, Arrowhead Mills	¼ cup	0/1
Hamburger buns, organic sprouted grain, Food for Life Ezekiel 4:9	1	0/2
Hamburger buns, sprouted grain, sesame, Food for Life Ezekiel 4:9	1	0/2
Hot dog buns, 100% whole wheat, Oroweat	1	2/2
Hot dog buns, sprouted grain, Food for Life Ezekiel 4:9	1	0/2
Muffin, banana nut, VitaMuffin, Vitalicious	1	0/2
Taco shell, baked, 5"	1	0/1
Tortilla, brown rice, Food for Life	1	0/2
Tortilla, fajita, carb balance, whole wheat, Mission, 6"	1	0/1
Tortilla, low-carb/low-fat, large size, La Tortilla Factory	1	1/1
Tortilla, low-fat, Smart & Delicious, La Tortilla Factory	1	1/2
Tortilla, Smart & Delicious, La Tortilla Factory	1	1/1
Tortilla, sprouted grain, corn, Food for Life	2	1/2
Tortilla, sprouted grain, Food for Life Ezekiel 4:9	1	0/2
Tortilla, white corn, Mission, 6"	1	0/1

9. PASTA

FOOD ITEM	SERVING	S/C VALUE
Pasta, angel hair, Barilla Plus, Barilla	2 oz.	2/2
Pasta, fettuccine, sprouted grain, Food for Life Ezekiel 4:9	2 oz.	0/2
Pasta, penne, Barilla Plus, Barilla	2 oz.	2/2
Pasta, penne, sprouted grain, Food for Life Ezekiel 4:9	2 oz.	2/2
Pasta, rotini, Barilla Plus, Barilla	2 oz.	2/2
Pasta, spaghetti, sprouted grain, Food for Life Ezekiel 4:9	2 oz.	0/2
Pasta, veggie spirals, Wacky Mac	2 oz.	0/3

10. CEREAL & GRAINS

FOOD ITEM	SERVING	S/C VALUE
Cereal, buckwheat, hot	2 Tbsp.	0/2
Cereal, cornflakes	½ cup	1/1
Cereal, corn flakes, U.S. Mills Erewhon	1 cup	0/2
Cereal, cream of rice, cooked	½ cup	0/1
Cereal, crispy brown rice, gluten free, U.S. Mills Erewhon	1 cup	0/2
Cereal, crispy brown rice with mixed berries, U.S. Mills Erewhon	1 cup	0/2
Cereal, Fiber One, General Mills	½ cup	0/2
Cereal, Grape-Nuts, Post	¾ cup	4/3
Cereal, Grape-Nuts Flakes, Post	½ cup	4/2
Cereal, oat-bran flakes	¾ cup	6/2
Cereal, oatmeal, old-fashioned, dry	¼ cup	1/1
Cereal, puffed rice	½ cup	0/1
Cereal, puffed wheat	½ cup	0/1
Cereal, puffs, whole grain, Kashi	1 cup	0/1
Cereal, Rice Chex, General Mills	½ cup	1/1
Cereal, Rice Krispies, Kellogg's	½ cup	1/1
Cereal, Shredded Wheat, Post	1 cup	0/2
Cereal, Shredded Wheat, spoon size, Post	⅓ cup	0/1
Cereal, Special K, Kellogg's	½ cup	2/1
Cereal, toasted oats, Cheerios, General Mills	1 cup	1/1
Cereal, Total, General Mills	½ cup	3/1
Cereal, Uncle Sam	⅓ cup	0/1
Cereal, Wheaties, General Mills	½ cup	1/1
Cereal, whole-grain, almond, Food for Life Ezekiel 4:9	½ cup	0/2
Cereal, whole grain, Food for Life Ezekiel 4:9	½ cup	0/2
Cereal, whole-grain, golden flax, Food for Life Ezekiel 4:9	½ cup	0/2
Cereal, whole-grain, original, Food for Life Ezekiel 4:9	½ cup	0/2
Cereal, whole-wheat, Uncle Sam, U.S. Mills	¾ cup	0/2
Couscous, plain, cooked	⅓ cup	0/1
Cream of Wheat, instant, B&G	1 pkt.	0/1
Flour, soy, Arrowhead Mills	¼ cup	0/1

FOOD ITEM	SERVING	S/C VALUE	FOOD ITEM	SERVING	S/C VALUE
Oatmeal, instant, U.S. Mills Uncle Sam	1 pkt.	0/2	Endive, head	½	1/1
Oatmeal, Irish, steel cut, McCann's	¼ cup	0/2	Fennel, bulb, sliced	1 cup	0/1
Oatmeal, quick 1-minute, Quaker	½ cup	1/1	Garlic, clove	1	0/0
Oatmeal, regular, instant, Quaker	1 pkt.	0/1	Ginger root, grated	1 tsp.	0/0
Rice, basmati, cooked	¼ cup	1/2	Grape leaves	1 cup	1/0
Rice, brown, long-grain, cooked	¼ cup	0/1	Green beans, cooked	1 cup	2/1
Rice, jasmine, cooked	¼ cup	0/1	Jalapeño pepper	1	0/0
Rice, long grain & wild, cooked, Uncle Ben's	½ cup	0/2	Jicama (yam bean), chopped	½ cup	1/1
Rice, Mexican fiesta, cooked, Uncle Ben's	½ cup	0/2	Kale, chopped, cooked	1 cup	2/1
Rice, quinoa, cooked	¼ cup	0/1	Leeks, chopped, raw	1 cup	4/1
Rice, white, long-grain, cooked	¼ cup	0/1	Lettuce, Bibb, large leaves	4	1/0
Rice, wild, cooked	¼ cup	0/1	Lettuce, Boston, medium leaves	4	0/0
Risotto, dry	2 Tbsp.	0/1	Lettuce, butterhead, leaves	4	0/0
			Lettuce, iceberg, large leaves	4	1/0
11. VEGETABLES			Lettuce, red leaf, inner leaves	4	0/0
Artichoke, medium	1	1/1	Lettuce, romaine, leaves	4	1/0
Artichoke hearts, marinated, Progresso	2	1/0	Mushrooms, brown, Italian, sliced	1 cup	1/0
Arugula	½ cup	0/0	Mushrooms, porcini, dried, pieces	4	1/0
Asparagus spears, cooked	4	1/0	Mushrooms, portobello, grilled	3 oz.	0/1
Bamboo shoots	½ cup	0/0	Mushrooms, shiitake	5	3/1
Bell pepper, green, raw, medium	1	3/1	Okra, cooked	1 cup	2/0
Bell pepper, red, raw, medium	1	5/1	Onion, green (scallion), chopped	¼ cup	1/0
Bell pepper, yellow, raw, medium	1	5/1	Onion, pearl, cooked	½ cup	4/1
Bok choy, cooked	1 cup	1/0	Onion, red, chopped	½ cup	4/1
Broccoflower, steamed	1 cup	0/1	Onion, red, large, slice	1	1/0
Broccoli, Chinese, cooked	1 cup	1/0	Onion, yellow, chopped	½ cup	3/1
Broccoli, florets	1 cup	2/0	Onion, yellow, large, slice	1	2/0
Brussels sprouts, cooked, drained, with salt	1 cup	3/1	Palm, hearts	1 oz.	0/1
Cabbage, shredded, cooked, with salt, drained	½ cup	2/0	Parsley, chopped	1 Tbsp.	0/0
Cabbage, shredded, raw	½ cup	1/0	Parsnips, cooked with salt	½ cup	4/1
Carrot, medium, raw	1	3/1	Peas, green, cooked	½ cup	4/1
Carrots, chopped, raw	½ cup	3/1	Peas, snow, steamed	½ cup	3/1
Cauliflower florets, raw	1 cup	1/1	Pepper, ancho, dried	1	0/1
Celery stalk, medium	1	0/0	Pepper, banana	1	1/0
Chicory root, raw	1 root	0/1	Pepper, hot chili, green	1	2/0
Cilantro, chopped	¼ cup	0/0	Pepper, hot chili, red	1	2/0
Collard greens, chopped, cooked	1 cup	1/1	Pepper, hot chili, sun dried	1	1/0
Corn, sweet, white	½ cup	3/1	Pepper, hot green, chopped	¼ cup	2/0
Corn, sweet, white, medium ear	1	3/2	Pepper, jalapeño	1	0/0
Corn, sweet, yellow	½ cup	2/1	Pepper, pasilla, dried	1	0/1
Corn, sweet, yellow, medium ear	1	3/2	Pickles, dill, Snack'mms, Vlasic	3	1/0
Cucumber, whole, 8"	1	4/1	Potato, baked, with skin, large	1	4/4
Eggplant, cubed, cooked	1 cup	3/1	Potato, russet, Steam n' Mash, Ore-Ida	¾ cup	0/1

FOOD ITEM	SERVING	S/C VALUE	FOOD ITEM	SERVING	S/C VALUE
Potato, diced with onion, frozen,	2/3 cup	0/1	Turnip, cubed	1 cup	5/1
Simply Potatoes			Vegetables blend, Normandy style,	3/4 cup	3/1
Potato, fingerling	1/2 cup	0/1	Kirkland Signature		
Potato, fries, shoe string, Cascadian Farm	3 oz.	1/2	Wasabi	1 tsp.	0/0
Potato, fries, steak cut, Ore-Ida	7	1/1	Water chestnuts, Chinese, canned	1/2 cup	3/1
Potato, hash browns, frozen, Cascadian Farm	1/2 cup	0/1	Watercress, chopped	1 cup	0/0
Potato, mashed, garlic seasoned,	3/4 cup	0/1	Yam, cooked	1/2 cup	0/1
Steam n' Mash, Ore-Ida			Zucchini, sliced	1 cup	3/1
Potato, mashed, three cheese, Steam n' Mash,	3/4 cup	0/1			
Ore-Ida					
Potato, red, baked, with skin, medium	1	3/2	## 12. FRUITS		
Potato, sweet, baked, large	1	10/2	Apple, Fuji	1/2	7/1
Potato, sweet, baked, without skin, large	1	15/2	Apple, Granny Smith, medium	1/2	7/1
Pumpkin, canned, with salt	1/2 cup	4/1	Apple, red delicious, medium	1/2	7/1
Radicchio, shredded	1 cup	0/0	Apricot, medium	1	3/0
Radishes, sliced, red	1/2 cup	1/0	Avocado	1/4 cup	0/0
Rutabaga, cubed	1/2 cup	5/1	Banana, medium	1/2	7/1
Sauerkraut, canned, low sodium	1 cup	3/1	Bananas, dried	1 oz.	10/1
Seaweed, nori	1/4 cup	0/0	Blackberries	1/2 cup	4/1
Shallots, chopped	1/4 cup	1/1	Blueberries	1/4 cup	4/1
Snap beans, green	1 cup	2/1	Cantaloupe, wedge	1	6/1
Snap beans, yellow	1 cup	2/1	Cherries, bing	8	7/1
Spinach, baby	1 cup	0/0	Cranberries, dried	2 Tbsp.	10/1
Spinach, raw	3 oz.	0/0	Grapefruit, red & pink, medium	1/2	9/1
Sprouts, alfalfa	1/4 cup	0/0	Grapes, red or green	1.7 oz.	8/1
Sprouts, bean	1/4 cup	1/0	Honeydew, wedge	1	10/1
Squash, acorn, cubed, cooked	2/3 cup	2/1	Kiwi, no skin, medium	1	7/1
Squash, butternut, cubed, cooked	1/2 cup	2/1	Lemon, wedge	1	0/0
Squash, crookneck, slices, cooked, with salt	1/2 cup	2/0	Lime, wedge	1	0/0
Squash, hubbard, cubed, cooked	1/2 cup	1/1	Mango, sliced	1/2 cup	12/1
Squash, scallop, sliced, cooked, with salt	1/2 cup	1/0	Nectarine, sliced	1/2 cup	5/1
Squash, spaghetti, baked	1/2 cup	2/1	Olives, black	.5 oz.	0/0
Squash, straightneck, sliced	1/2 cup	2/0	Olives, green, Castella	.6 oz.	0/0
Squash, summer, sliced, cooked, with salt	1/2 cup	1/0	Olives, Kalamata, Castella	.5 oz.	0/0
Squash, winter, cubed	1/2 cup	2/1	Orange, small	1	9/1
Swiss chard, chopped, cooked	1 cup	0/0	Peach, sliced, medium	1	7/1
Taro, cooked	1/4 cup	0/1	Pear	1/2	7/1
Tomatillo, chopped	1/2 cup	3/0	Pineapple, diced	1/2 cup	7/1
Tomatoes, cherry, red	1 cup	4/1	Plum, medium	1	7/1
Tomatoes, grape	1 cup	4/1	Raspberries	1/2 cup	3/1
Tomatoes, red, chopped	1 cup	5/1	Rhubarb, diced	1 cup	1/1
Tomatoes, red, diced, canned, without salt	1/2 cup	4/1	Strawberry	1/2 cup	4/1
Tomatoes, red, sliced, medium	1	1/0	Tangerine, medium	1	9/1
			Watermelon, diced	1 cup	9/1

FOOD ITEM	SERVING	S/C VALUE
13. SWEETENERS		
Honey substitute, Tastes Like Honey, Nature's Hollow	1 Tbsp.	0/1
Honey, Raw	1 Tbsp.	16/1
Natural sweetener, PureVia	1 pkt.	0/0
Natural sweetener, Stevia Extract in the Raw	1 pkt.	0/0
Natural sweetener, Stevia	1 pkt.	0/0
Natural sweetener, Sweet Fiber	1 pkt.	0/0
Natural sweetener, Sweet Simplicity	1 pkt.	0/1
Natural sweetener, Truvia	1 pkt.	0/0
Natural sweetener, Xylitol Crystals	1 pkt.	0/0
Natural sweetener, xylitol packets, NOW Foods	1 pkt.	0/0
Natural sweetener, xylitol packets, Xlear, Inc. XyloSweet	1 pkt.	0/0
Natural sweetener, Xlear, Inc. XyloSweet	1 tsp.	0/0
Natural sweetener, ZSweet	1 tsp.	0/0
Sweetener, maltitol, Joseph's	¼ cup	0/1
Sugar, pure cane, white granulated, C&H	1 tsp.	4/0
Sugar, Sugar in the Raw	1 pkt.	4/0
14. OILS		
Almond oil	1 Tbsp.	0/0
Avocado oil	1 Tbsp.	0/0
Butter, with salt	1 Tbsp.	0/0
Canola oil	1 Tbsp.	0/0
Coconut oil, Barlean's	1 Tbsp.	0/0
Codfish oil	1 Tbsp.	0/0
Cooking spray, olive oil, Pam	⅓ sec.	0/0
Flax oil, Barlean's	1 Tbsp.	0/0
Flax oil, highest lignan, Barlean's	1 Tbsp.	0/0
Hemp oil, Living Harvest	2 Tbsp.	0/0
Olive oil, dipping oil, herb-flavored, Annie's Naturals	1 Tbsp.	0/0
	1 Tbsp.	0/0
Olive oil, extra virgin, Kirkland Signature		
Olive oil, extra virgin, Rachael Ray	1 Tbsp.	0/0
Omega Swirl, lemon zest, Barlean's	2 tsp.	0/0
Omega Swirl, pomegranate blueberry, Barlean's	1 Tbsp.	0/0
Omega Swirl, strawberry banana, Barlean's	1 Tbsp.	0/1
Sesame Oil	1 Tbsp.	0/0
Vegetable Oil	1 Tbsp.	0/0
15. SNACKS		
Almonds, smokehouse, Blue Diamond	1 oz.	1/0

FOOD ITEM	SERVING	S/C VALUE
Almonds, bold jalapeño smokehouse, Blue Diamond	1 oz.	1/1
Almonds, dry roasted, without salt	.5 oz.	1/0
Almonds, Kirkland Signature	1 oz.	1/1
Almonds, oven roasted, sliced, original, Sunkist	.5 oz.	0/0
Bar, high protein, KETOslim, Nature's Plus	1	2/2
Brazil nuts	1 oz.	1/0
Brazil nuts, raw, Bates Nut Farm	1 oz.	1/0
Cashews, dry roasted, without salt	1 oz.	1/0
Cheddar puffs, baked, Garden of Eatin'	1 oz.	1/1
Cheese puffs, jumbo, Cheetos	1 oz.	1/1
Chips, cheddar & sour cream, Ruffles	1 oz.	0/1
Chips, cool ranch, Doritos	1 oz.	0/1
Chips, extreme blazin' buffalo wing, Pringles	1 oz.	0/1
Chips, krinkle cut, classic barbeque, Kettle Brand	1 oz.	1/1
Chips, lightly salted, Kettle Brand	1 oz.	0/1
Chips, lightly salted, krinkle cut, Kirkland Signature Kettle Brand	1 oz.	0/1
Chips, nacho cheese, Doritos	1 oz.	1/1
Chips, natural blue corn, Tostitos	1 oz.	0/1
Chips, original corn chips, Fritos	1 oz.	0/1
Chips, original, Pringles	1 oz.	0/1
Chips, pita, parmesan garlic & herb, Stacy's Simply Naked	1 oz.	0/1
Chips, restaurant style tortilla triangles, Mission	1 oz.	0/1
Chips, sea salt & vinegar, Kettle Brand	1 oz.	0/1
Chips, spicy salsa tortilla rounds, Salsitas, El Sabroso	1 oz.	0/1
Chips, tortilla rounds, Mission	1 oz.	0/1
Chips, tortilla triangles, Mission	10	0/1
Chips, wavy hickory BBQ, Lay's	1 oz.	0/1
Chips, yogurt & green onion, Kettle Brand	1 oz.	0/1
Corn snack, aged white cheddar, Pirate's Booty	1 oz.	0/1
Corn snack, Pirate's Booty	1 oz.	0/1
Corn snack, barbeque, Pirate's Booty	1 oz.	0/1
Corn snack, Bermuda onion, Pirate's Booty	1 oz.	0/1
Corn snack, sea salt & vinegar, Pirate's Booty	1 oz.	0/1
Corn snack, veggie, Pirate's Booty	1 oz.	0/1
Corn snack, Smart Puffs	1 oz.	0/1
Corn sticks, Original Tings	1 oz.	0/1
Crackers, better cheddars, Nabisco	22	0/1
Crackers, cheddar bunnies, Annie's Homegrown	50	0/1

FOOD ITEM	SERVING	S/C VALUE
Crackers, cheddar, goldfish, Pepperidge Farm	55	0/1
Crackers, Cheez-It, Sunshine	27	0/1
Crackers, crispbread, hearty rye, Wasa	1	0/1
Crackers, crispbread, multi grain, Wasa	1	0/1
Crackers, hot & spicy, Cheez-It, Sunshine	25	0/1
Crackers, klassic 3 seed flatbreads, Doctor Kracker	1 slice	0/1
Crackers, 100-calorie pack, Ritz snack mix, Nabisco	1 pkg.	2/1
Crackers, seasoned, RyKrisp	2	0/1
Crackers, table water, Carr's	5 ea.	0/1
Crackers, Triscuit, Nabisco	.75 oz.	0/1
Jerky, beef, plain, large	.7 oz.	0/0
Jerky, beef, teriyaki, Oh Boy! Oberto	1 oz.	5/1
Mixed nuts, Emerald	1 oz.	1/1
Mixed nuts, nuts & dried fruit, Eden Selected All Mixed Up	1.1 oz.	2/1
Peanuts, dry roasted, without salt	1 oz.	1/0
Pecan, halves, Kirkland Signature	1 oz.	1/0
Pecans	1 oz.	1/0
Pine nuts, Kirkland Signature	1 oz.	1/0
Pistachios	10 ea.	1/0
Popcorn, air popped	1 cup	0/1
Popcorn, hall of fame kettle corn, Dale and Thomas Popcorn	½ cup	6/1
Popcorn, microwave, reduced sodium	.5 oz.	0/1
Popcorn, popped, butter lover's, Act II	4 cups	0/1
Popcorn, popped, kettle corn, Act II	1 cup	0/1
Popcorn, unpopped, old fashioned butter, Orville Redenbacher's	2 Tbsp.	0/1
Popcorn, unpopped, tender white, Orville Redenbacher's	2 Tbsp.	0/1
Pretzels, classic style, tiny twists, Rold Gold	1 oz.	1/2
Pretzels, honey mustard & onion nibblers, Snyder's of Hanover	1 oz.	1/2
Puffs, Cheetos	1 oz.	1/1
Pumpkin seeds, dry roasted, Eden Organic	¼ cup	0/0
Rice cakes, mini, buttered popcorn, Quaker	1 pkg.	0/1
Rice cakes, plain, unsalted	1 ea.	0/0
Salmon, cups, Chicken of the Sea	1 cup	0/0
Snack bar, chocolate brownie, Doctor's CarbRite	1 bar	0/2
Snack mix, chex mix, General Mills	1 oz.	2/2
Soup, chicken noodle, Healthy Choice	½ can	0/1
Soup, chicken with rice, Healthy Choice	½ can	0/1

FOOD ITEM	SERVING	S/C VALUE
Soy nuts, roasted, Emerald	¼ cup	0/1
Sunflower seeds, It's Delish!	1 oz.	1/1
Tuna, cups, Chicken of the Sea	1 cup	0/0
Veggie stix, Good Health Natural Products	1 oz.	0/1
Walnuts, black, dried, chopped	1 oz.	1/0
Walnuts, Kirkland Signature	1 oz.	1/0

16. TREATS

FOOD ITEM	SERVING	S/C VALUE
Brownies, pecan walnut, sugar-free, Joseph's	4	0/1
Cakes, chocolate raspberry, sugar-free, Joseph's	4	0/1
Candies, berry, Xlear, Inc. SparX	1	0/0
Candies, citrus, Xlear, Inc. SparX	1	0/0
Candies, fruit, Xlear Inc. SparX	1	0/0
Caramels, vanilla, sugar free, Judy's Candy Company	1	0/1
Chocolate, baking cocoa, unsweetened, Hershey's	1 Tbsp.	0/0
Chocolate, bar, Belgian milk chocolate, raspberry, La Nouba	1	0/2
Chocolate, bar, dark chocolate, ChocoPerfection, LowCarb Specialties, Inc.	1	0/1
Chocolate, bar, dark, organic, Green & Black's	⅓	5/1
Chocolate, bar, milk chocolate, ChocoPerfection, LowCarb Specialties, Inc.	1	0/1
Chocolate, bar, milk, low effective carb & sugar free, Carb Safe, D-lectable	¼	2/1
Chocolate chips, sugar free, Hershey's	1 Tbsp.	0/1
Chocolate, dark, peppermint patties, sugar free, York	3	0/2
Chocolate drink, kidz superfood, Amazing Grass	1 scoop	0/0
Chocolate, marshmallow, La Nouba	1	0/1
Chocolate, pieces, dark, sugar free, Dove	5	0/2
Chocolate, pieces, extreme dark chocolate, Endangered Species Chocolate	4	5/1
Chocolates, sugar free, Hershey's	5	0/2
Cinna cubs, sugar free, Perfectly Sweet	9	0/2
Cookies, almond, sugar-free, Joseph's	4	0/1
Cookies, chocolate chip, sugar-free, Joseph's	4	0/1
Cookies, chocolate mint, sugar-free, Joseph's	4	0/1
Cookies, chocolate peanut butter, sugar-free, Joseph's	4	0/1
Cookies, chocolate walnut, sugar-free, Joseph's	4	0/1
Cookies, coconut macaroons, unsweetened,	2	1/1

FOOD ITEM	SERVING	S/C VALUE
Jennies		
Cookies, coconut, sugar-free, Joseph's	4	0/1
Cookies, crunchy granola, triple nut,	1	5/1
Pepperidge Farm		
Cookies, lemon, sugar-free, Joseph's	4	0/1
Cookies, oatmeal chocolate chip with pecans,	4	0/1
sugar-free, Joseph's		
Cookies, oatmeal, sugar-free, Joseph's	4	0/1
Cookies, 100-calorie pack, chessmen,	1 pkg.	5/1
Pepperidge Farm		
Cookies, peanut butter, sugar-free, Joseph's	4	0/1
Cookies, pecan chocolate chip, sugar-free, Joseph's	4	0/1
Cookies, pecan shortbread, sugar-free, Joseph's	4	0/1
Corn snack, Pirate's Booty	1 oz.	0/1
Gum, cinnamon, Xlear, Inc. Spry	1	0/0
Gum, fresh fruit, Xlear, Inc. Spry	1	0/0
Gum, green tea, Xlear, Inc. Spry	1	0/0
Gum, peppermint, Xlear, Inc. Spry	1	0/0
Gum, spearmint, Xlear, Inc. Spry	1	0/0
Hard candy, sugar free, Jolly Rancher	4	0/1
Licorice, strawberry, sugar free vines, Red Vines	7	0/2
Licorice, twists, black, sugar free, Perfectly Sweet	7	0/2
Licorice, twists, strawberry, sugar free vines,	7	0/2
Red Vines		
Mints, berryblast, Xlear, Inc. Spry	1	0/0
Mints, lemonburst, Xlear, Inc. Spry	1	0/0
Mints, power peppermints, Xlear, Inc. Spry	1	0/0
Muffin, sugar free, velvety chocolate, VitaMuffin,	1	0/2
Vitalicious		
Muffin top, sugar free, velvety chocolate,	1	0/2
VitaTop, Vitalicious		
Omega Swirl, chocolate raspberry, Barlean's	1 Tbsp.	0/1
Omega Swirl, lemon zest, Barlean's	2 tsp.	0/0
Omega Swirl, orange cream, Barlean's	1 Tbsp.	0/1
Omega Swirl, pomegranate blueberry, Barlean's	1 Tbsp.	0/1
Omega Swirl, strawberry banana, Barlean's	1 Tbsp.	0/1
Peanut brittle, sugar free, Judy's Candy	¾ cup	0/1
Company		
Sauce, pecan praline, sugar free,	2 Tbsp.	0/1
Perfectly Sweet		
Whipped topping, nonfat, 365 Everyday Value	2 Tbsp.	0/0

17. BEVERAGES & POWDERED DRINKS

FOOD ITEM	SERVING	S/C VALUE
Beer, Bud Light	12 oz.	0/1
Beer, Coors Light	12 oz.	0/1
Beer, Michelob Ultra	12 oz.	0/0
Beer, Miller Chill	12 oz.	0/0
Beer, Miller Lite	12 oz.	0/0
Beer, non-alcoholic, O'Doul's	12 oz.	0/1
Champagne, extra dry, Korbel	4 oz.	0/0
Club soda, Canada Dry	8 oz.	0/0
Coffee, black (any size)	6 oz.	0/0
Coffee, classic decaf, Folgers	2 Tbsp.	0/0
Coffee, classic roast, Folgers	2 Tbsp.	0/0
Coffee, decaf, Nescafé clasico, Nescafé	2 Tbsp.	0/0
Coffee, house blend, Kirkland Signature	2 Tbsp.	0/0
Coffee, house blend, Starbucks	2 Tbsp.	0/0
Iced-tea drink, unsweetened, Tejava	8 oz.	0/0
Juice drink, True Lemon	1 pkt.	0/0
Nutrition drink, kidz superfood outrageous	1 scoop	1/0
chocolate flavor, Amazing Grass		
Protein drink, whey, chocolate, Jay Robb	1 scoop	0/0
Protein drink, whey, piña colada, Jay Robb	1 scoop	0/0
Protein drink, whey, strawberry, Jay Robb	1 scoop	0/0
Protein drink, whey, tropical dreamsicle, Jay Robb	1 scoop	0/0
Protein drink, whey, vanilla, Jay Robb	1 scoop	0/0
Soda, natural black cherry, Zevia	12 oz.	0/1
Soda, natural cola, Zevia	12 oz.	0/1
Soda, natural ginger ale, Zevia	12 oz.	0/1
Soda, natural orange, Zevia	12 oz.	0/1
Soda, natural twist, Zevia	12 oz.	0/1
Soda, natural root beer, Zevia	12 oz.	0/1
Soymilk, plain, Silk	1 cup	6/1
Sports drink, Propel Fit Water, Gatorade	8 oz.	2/0
Tea bag, black, Bavarian wild berry, Lipton	1	0/0
Tea bag, green tea with mandarin orange flavor,	1	0/0
Lipton		
Tea bag, red tea with harvest strawberry	1	0/0
& passionfruit flavor, Lipton		
Tea bag, black, Tuscan lemon, Lipton	1	0/0
Tea bag, white tea with blueberry & pomegranate	1	0/0
flavor, Lipton		
Tea bag, white tea with island mango & peach	1	0/0
flavors, Lipton		

FOOD ITEM	SERVING	S/C VALUE
Tea bag, 100% natural green tea, Lipton	1	0/0
Tea bag, bedtime story herbal tea, Lipton	1	0/0
Tea bag, black pearl, Lipton	1	0/0
Tea, green tea, matcha blend, Kirkland Signature	1	0/0
Tea, green, Bigelow	1	0/0
Tea bag, French vanilla, Lipton		0/0
Tea bag, iced tea mix, unsweetened, decaffeinated, Lipton	2 Tbsp.	0/0
Tea drink, passionfruit, The Republic of Tea	1	0/1
Tea drink, pomegranate, The Republic of Tea	1	0/0
Tea, unsweetened plain, hot or iced (any size)	8 oz.	0/0
Tea bag, vanilla caramel truffle, Lipton	1	0/0
Vitamin/energy drink, berry, Amazing Grass	1 scoop	0/0
Vitamin/energy drink, chocolate, Amazing Grass	1 scoop	0/0
Vitamin/energy drink, lemonade, Ultima Replenisher	1 pkt.	0/0
Vitamin/energy drink, pink lemonade	1 pkt.	0/0
Vitamin/energy drink, source of life bright lightning, Nature's Plus	2 tsp.	1/1
Vitamin/energy drink, source of life red lightning, Nature's Plus	2 tsp.	1/1
Vitamin/energy drink, orange, Ultima Replenisher	1 pkt.	0/0
Vitamin/energy drink, wild raspberry, Ultima Replenisher	1 pkt.	0/0
Water, black and blue berry, lifewater, SoBe	20 oz.	0/1
Water, fuji apple pear, lifewater, SoBe	20 oz.	0/1
Water, Kirkland Signature	20 oz.	0/0
Water, plain	8 oz.	0/0
Water, sparkling	8 oz.	0/0
Water, sparkling, lemon, Perrier	8 oz.	0/0
Water, sparkling, S.Pellegrino	8 oz.	0/0
Water, yumberry pomegranate, lifewater, SoBe	20 oz.	0/1
Wheat grass, Amazing Grass	1 Tbsp.	0/0
White wine, chardonnay, Kendall-Jackson	5 oz.	0/0
White wine, chardonnay, Kirkland Signature	5 oz.	0/0
Wine, champagne	4 oz.	0/0
Wine, dessert	3.5 oz.	8/1
Wine, red	5 oz.	0/1
Wine, red, cabernet sauvignon, J. Lohr	5 oz.	0/1
Wine, red, cabernet sauvignon, Kirkland Signature	5 oz.	0/1

18. SAUCES, CONDIMENTS & DRESSINGS

FOOD ITEM	SERVING	S/C VALUE
Almond butter, MaraNatha	2 Tbsp.	2/1
Anchovy paste, Alessi	1 Tbsp.	0/0
Barbecue sauce, hickory maple, Nature's Hollow	2 Tbsp.	0/0
Barbecue sauce, honey mustard, Nature's Hollow	1 Tbsp.	0/0
Barbecue sauce, Scott's	1 Tbsp.	0/0
Black pepper, Kirkland Signature	1 Tbsp.	0/0
Cinnamon, ground, highland harvested Saigon, The Spice Hunter	1 tsp.	0/0
Dressing, Caesar, Newman's Own	2 Tbsp.	1/0
Dressing, cowgirl ranch, Annie's Naturals	2 Tbsp.	2/0
Dressing, Italian, restaurant recipe, Bernstein's	2 Tbsp.	0/0
Dressing, oil and vinegar, Lighten Up, Newman's Own	2 Tbsp.	2/0
Dressing, oil and vinegar, Newman's Own	2 Tbsp.	1/0
Dressing, ranch, Newman's Own	2 Tbsp.	1/0
Dressing, vinaigrette, balsamic, Lighten Up, Newman's Own	2 Tbsp.	1/0
Dressing, vinaigrette, balsamic, Newman's Own	2 Tbsp.	1/0
Dressing, vinaigrette, shiitake & sesame, Annie's Naturals	2 Tbsp.	1/0
Enchilada sauce, green, La Victoria	¼ cup	0/0
Enchilada sauce, red, La Victoria	¼ cup	0/0
Enchilada sauce, red chile sauce, La Victoria	¼ cup	0/0
Gravy, rich mushroom, Heinz	¼ cup	0/0
Gravy, savory beef, Heinz	¼ cup	0/0
Guacamole, Wholly Guacamole	2 Tbsp.	0/0
Hot sauce, Tabasco Pepper Sauce	1 tsp.	0/0
Hummus, roasted red peppers, all-natural, Tribe	2 Tbsp.	0/0
Jam, raspberry, sugar free, Nature's Hollow	1 Tbsp.	0/1
Jam, wild blueberry, sugar free, Nature's Hollow	1 Tbsp.	0/1
Ketchup, organic, Heinz	1 Tbsp.	4/0
Ketchup, sugar free, Nature's Hollow	1 Tbsp.	0/1
Mayonnaise with olive oil, Kraft	2 Tbsp.	0/0
Mayonnaise, Best Foods	2 Tbsp.	0/0
Mayonnaise, hot & spicy, Kraft	1 Tbsp.	0/0
Mayonnaise, Kraft	1 Tbsp.	0/0
Miracle Whip, light, Kraft	2 Tbsp.	2/0
Mustard, chipotle, Silver Springs	1 tsp.	0/0
Mustard, classic yellow, French's	1 tsp.	0/0
Mustard, dijon, Grey Poupon	1 Tbsp.	0/0
Mustard, kicked up horseradish, Emeril's	1 tsp.	0/0

FOOD ITEM	SERVING	S/C VALUE
Mustard, spicy brown, French's	1 tsp.	0/0
Pasta sauce, family marinara, Amy's	½ cup	5/1
Pasta sauce, marinara di Venezia, Seeds of Change	½ cup	0/1
Pasta sauce, roasted garlic, DeLallo	½ cup	1/1
Pasta sauce, Romagna three cheese, Seeds of Change	½ cup	0/1
Pasta sauce, tomato basil Genovese, Seeds of Change	½ cup	0/1
Pasta sauce, vodka Americana, Seeds of Change	½ cup	1/1
Peanut butter, creamy, sugar-free, Joseph's	2 Tbsp.	0/1
Peanut butter, crunchy, sugar-free, Joseph's	2 Tbsp.	0/1
Peanut butter, Laura Scudder's	1.1 oz.	1/1
Peanut butter, organic, creamy, Kirkland Signature	2 Tbsp.	2/1
Peanut butter, natural, Skippy	2 Tbsp.	3/1
Pesto, basil, Classico	2 Tbsp.	1/0
Pesto, DeLallo	1 Tbsp.	0/0
Preserves, apricot, sugar free, Nature's Hollow	1 Tbsp.	0/1
Preserves, mountain berry, sugar free, Nature's Hollow	1 Tbsp.	0/1
Preserves, peach, sugar free, Nature's Hollow	1 Tbsp.	0/1
Preserves, raspberry, sugar free, Nature's Hollow	1 Tbsp.	0/1
Preserves, strawberry, sugar free, Nature's Hollow	1 Tbsp.	0/1
Preserves, wild blueberry, sugar free, Nature's Hollow	1 Tbsp.	0/1
Relish, dill, Heinz	1 Tbsp.	0/0
Salsa, Green Mountain Gringo	2 Tbsp.	0/0
Salsa, organic, Kirkland Signature	2 Tbsp.	1/0
Salsa, salsa suprema, La Victoria	1 Tbsp.	0/0
Salt, pink, Himalania	1 Tbsp.	0/0
Sauce, classic Alfredo, Ragú	¼ cup	0/0
Sauce, creamy Alfredo, Classico	¼ cup	1/0
Sauce, pizza, Ragú	¼ cup	3/0
Soy sauce, less sodium, Kikkoman	1 Tbsp.	0/0
Syrup, caramel, Seelect Tea	2 Tbsp.	0/1
Syrup, maple, sugar free, Joseph's	2 Tbsp.	0/0
Syrup, maple, sugar free, Nature's Hollow	¼ cup	0/1
Syrup, raspberry, sugar free, Nature's Hollow	¼ cup	0/1
Taco sauce, green, La Victoria	2 Tbsp.	0/0
Tahini, roasted, sesame, MaraNatha	2 Tbsp.	0/1
Teriyaki sauce, Kikkoman	1 Tbsp.	2/0

FOOD ITEM	SERVING	S/C VALUE
Vinegar, balsamic	2 Tbsp.	0/0
Vinegar, malt, Heinz	1 Tbsp.	0/0
Vinegar, rice, Nakano, Mizkan	1 Tbsp.	0/0
Worcestershire, reduced sodium, French's	1 tsp.	0/0

19. FROZEN FOODS

Amy's Frozen Meals

Black Bean Vegetable Enchilada	1	2/2
Shepherd's Pie	1	5/2
Spinach Feta in a Pocket Sandwich	1	4/2
Mexican Tofu Scramble	1	5/2

Lean Cuisine Frozen Meals

Alfredo Pasta with Chicken & Broccoli	1	5/2
Baked Chicken	1	5/2
Baked Chicken Florentine	1	5/1
Beef Pot Roast	1	5/2
Chicken & Vegetables	1	5/2
Chicken Carbonara	1	5/2
Chicken Marsala	1	4/1
Chicken with Basil Cream Sauce	1	5/2
Chophouse Steak Flatbread Melts	1	4/2
Glazed Chicken	1	5/2
Grilled Chicken Caesar	1	2/2
Lemongrass Chicken	1	4/2
Meatloaf with Gravy & Whipped Potatoes	1	4/2
Roasted Chicken with Lemon Pepper Fettuccini	1	3/2
Roasted Garlic Chicken	1	3/1
Roasted Turkey & Vegetables	1	4/1
Rosemary Chicken	1	1/2
Salmon with Basil	1	3/2
Salmon Mediterranean	1	3/2
Salisbury Steak with Macaroni & Cheese	1	4/2
Shrimp Alfredo	1	5/2
Shrimp & Angel Hair Pasta	1	5/2
Steak Tips Portabello	1	4/1
Swedish Meatballs	1	4/2
Three Cheese Chicken	1	5/1

20. FAST FOOD/DINING OUT

Taco Bell

Cheese Quesadilla	1	4/2

FOOD ITEM	SERVING	S/C VALUE
Crunchy Taco	1	1/1
Fresco Crunchy Taco	1	1/1
Fresco Soft Taco–Beef	1	2/2
Grilled Steak Soft Taco	1	2/1
Nachos	1	3/2
Crunchy Taco Supreme	1	2/1
Tostada	1	2/2

McDonald's

FOOD ITEM	SERVING	S/C VALUE
Chipotle BBQ Snack Wrap (Crispy)	1	4/2
Chipotle BBQ Snack Wrap (Grilled)	1	5/2
Egg McMuffin	1	3/2
Ranch Snack Wrap (Crispy)	1	2/2
Ranch Snack Wrap (Grilled)	1	2/2

Rubio's

FOOD ITEM	SERVING	S/C VALUE
Chicken Taquitos	3	1/2
Enchilada, Chicken	1	2/2
Fish Taco Especial	1	4/2
Grilled Chicken Taco	1	2/2
Grilled Gourmet Taco, Steak	1	1/2
Grilled Steak Taco	1	1/2
HealthMex Chicken Taco	1	2/2
Street Taco, Steak	1	0/1

Subway Sandwiches

FOOD ITEM	SERVING	S/C VALUE
Black Forest Ham, Kids Pak Sandwich	1	4/2
Roast Beef, Kids Pak Sandwich	1	4/2
Tuna, 6"	1	5/3
Turkey Breast, Kids Pak Sandwich	1	4/2
Veggie Delite, 6"	1	6/3

Starbucks

FOOD ITEM	SERVING	S/C VALUE
Bacon, Gouda, Cheese, Egg Frittata on Artisan Roll	1	1/2
Chop Chop Pasta Salad	1	2/2
Rosemary Ham and Swiss Sandwich	1	2/2
Turkey & Swiss Sandwich	1	5/2

Kentucky Fried Chicken

FOOD ITEM	SERVING	S/C VALUE
Grilled Chicken Breast w/Mashed Potatoes, Gravy, and Green Beans	1	1/2
Grilled Chicken Wings (4) w/Mac & Cheese	1	4/1

Carl's Jr./Hardee's

FOOD ITEM	SERVING	S/C VALUE
Jumbo Chili Dog	1	4/2
Spicy Chicken Sandwich	1	3/2

Burger King

FOOD ITEM	SERVING	S/C VALUE
BK Double Stacker	1	5/2
Eight-Piece Crown-Shaped Chicken Tenders	1	0/2
Spicy Chick'n Crisp Sandwich	1	4/2

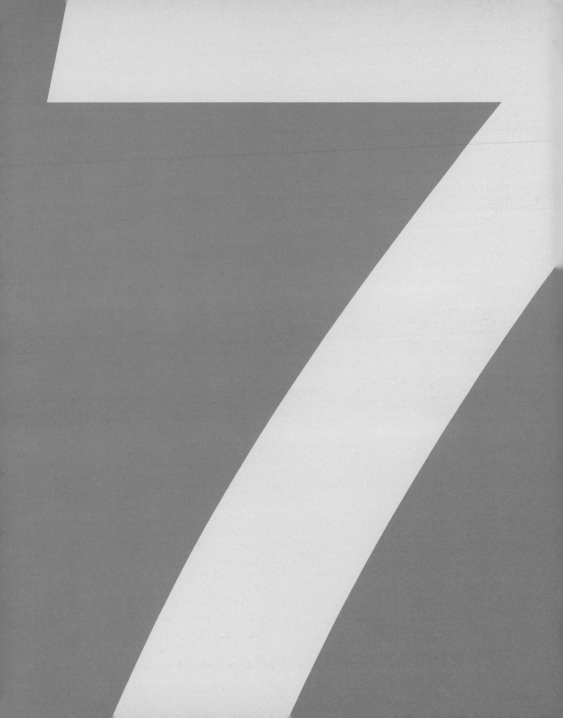

7

Tone Your
Abs

In this chapter, I'm going to show you a few of my secret tips for toning your abs once you've lost your belly fat. Keep in mind, though, that everything I cover in this chapter is completely optional. While the Belly Fat Cure doesn't require any exercise at all to lose up to 4 pounds a week, I'd like to encourage you to add some exercise into your daily life for overall toning and strength. To really enhance your midsection, I recommend this simple ab routine that I use every morning. I call it my 8-Minute Ab Sculptor.

Just follow the routine on the next page each morning after you wake up. The great thing is that it only takes about 8 minutes. There are three movements that work the top, bottom, and sides of your abdominals. I want you to do each exercise for approximately 30 seconds, then rest for 30 seconds, and then move right into the next exercise. After you've completed one round of all three exercises, rest 30 seconds, and repeat the entire sequence again so that each exercise in the series is performed twice.

WALKING

Another exercise I recommend for your overall health is walking. I suggest that you try to get in a 20-minute power walk as often as possible. When you power-walk for just 20 minutes, you improve your cardiovascular health and reduce stress.

The secret is to do it at the right intensity. To get that right intensity, make sure your heart rate is at 65 to 80 percent of your maximum rate. A simple method to determine this is the self-talk test. You accomplish this by walking at a challenging pace where you're breathing deeply and not gasping for air. On a treadmill for me, this is at an incline level of 12 and a 3.5 speed. Or you can imagine a scale of 0 to 10: 0 being when you're at rest, and 10 being when you're "all out" and gasping. Your goal is to aim for *a 6 to an 8* on the scale.

Remember, this is not essential to lose weight, but it will create an improved sense of well-being and boost your cardiovascular health.

8-MINUTE AB SCULPTOR

TOE REACH
Lie on your back. Cross your legs, flex your feet, and extend your legs into the air. With your arms extended and chin up, exhale as you crunch up, reaching toward your toes in a smooth, controlled motion. Squeeze and contract your abs at the top of the exercise, then inhale as you lower yourself back, never losing the tension on your abs and keeping your shoulder blades from touching the ground. Without resting, repeat for a total of 30 seconds, then rest for 30 seconds before moving on to the next exercise.

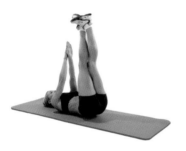 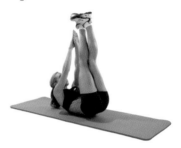

REVERSE CRUNCH
Lie on a mat with your hands by your sides, palms down. Pull your heels up as close to your butt as possible. Raise your heels up about two inches off the ground. Keep your chin up and abs tight. Exhale as you pull your knees up using the lower abdominals in a smooth, controlled motion. Squeeze and contract your abs at the top of the exercise (when your butt is off the ground). Then inhale as you lower yourself back, never losing the tension on your abs and keeping your shoulder blades from touching the ground. Without resting, repeat for a total of 30 seconds, then rest for 30 seconds before moving on to the next exercise.

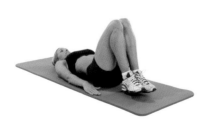 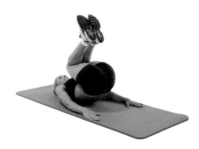

RUSSIAN TWIST

Sit on the mat with your knees bent, feet together. Keep your chin up and abs tight as you lean back slightly and lift your feet about two inches off the mat, engaging your abs. Extend your arms away from your chest with your palms pressed together, and turn to one side to begin the exercise. Exhale as you slowly rotate your torso as far as possible to the opposite side in a smooth, controlled motion. Squeeze and contract your abs. Inhale as you rotate back to the other side, keeping the tension on the abs. Without resting, repeat for a total of 30 seconds, then rest for 30 seconds before moving on to the next exercise.

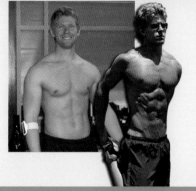

Jared lost 3 pounds

Age: 28
Height: 5'11"
Pounds Lost: 3
Belly Inches Lost: 2

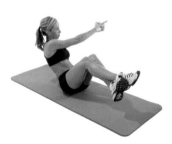

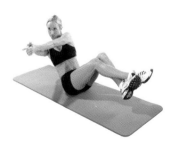

"As a fitness model, I am often asked this question, 'How do I get ripped?' In other words, people want to be able to see their abs 'pop.' I always tell them that based on my own personal success, the number one key without a doubt is not eating sugar and processed carbs. You can work out as hard and as much as you want, but 80 percent of your success lies in what you eat. Believe it—you can get ripped without any pills or drugs. I can say this because I've lived it, and that's why the Belly Fat Cure kicks butt."

BEST TIP FOR SUCCESS:

**"Preparing my meals in a specific pattern
and eating in that same pattern
every day, almost exactly like
Jorge's No-Excuses Day on page 25."**

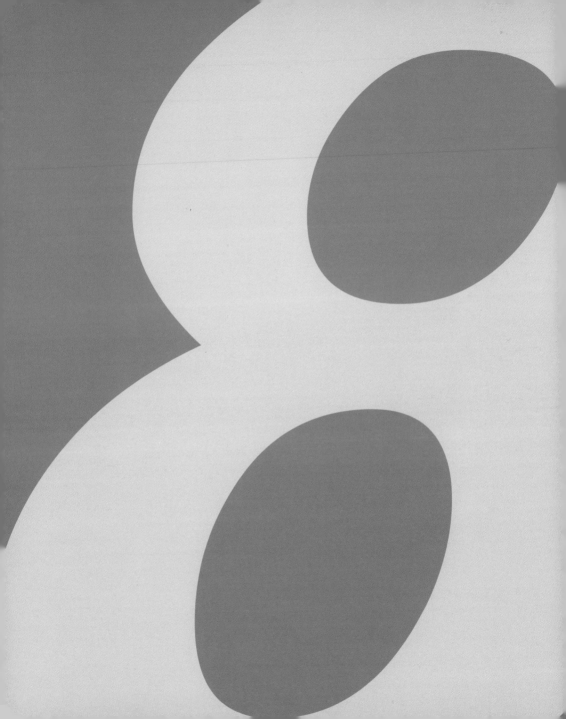

8 FAQs

1. **Does this plan work for everyone, regardless of age, gender, or body weight?**

   The Belly Fat Cure is a simple, eat-smarter solution that can absolutely work for everyone. I've had people from ages 16 to 100 follow this plan and lose the belly fat! My grandmother Maria, who is 100 years young, follows the plan and is so vital that she continues to live on her own. She has avoided sugar almost all of her life. And my two sons, Parker (five years old) and Owen (two years old), also follow this plan, and neither of them has been sick since they stopped drinking sugary milk or fruit drinks. Their favorite snacks are nuts, cheese, and low-sugar fruits. For your own children and teens, I recommend checking with your family doctor first. Keep in mind, though, that it's never too early to start monitoring sugar consumption; research has shown that even preschool-age kids are eating way too much of it. Since sugar doesn't have any nutritional benefits, its empty calories aren't good for anyone.

2. **Will this plan cost me a lot of money?**

   No. You can follow this plan simply by applying the S/C Value to your everyday eating. Check out page 25 for my "no excuses" basic eating day. It's inexpensive, easy, fast, and tasty! Of course, some of the foods I mention may be new to you, but they're completely optional. Keep in mind that when I recommend something new to you, it has been tested by me *personally* and was only granted my seal of approval because it tastes great.

3. **Do I have to exercise to lose belly fat?**

   No. Exercising is completely optional, and studies have shown that it can actually be counterproductive to weight loss. Research done at the University of Michigan revealed that typical forms of exercise don't burn enough calories to make a difference for weight-loss purposes. In fact, since it actually makes you hungrier, it can make eating the right amount of food each day difficult. Most of my clients in this book did not exercise at all to lose weight. However, once they lost their belly fat, many of them felt so good that they added exercise in and became addicted. When it's right for you, check out the strengthening and toning exercises in Chapter 7 or visit **JorgeCruise.com** for my other at-home plans.

4. **Do I have to starve myself?**

No way! This plan is not a diet. You're going to eat all the foods you love, including soda, chips, and ice cream. I'm just going to give you *smarter* options for enjoying all of these treats, *plus* great meals like four-cheese pizza, spaghetti with meat sauce, cheeseburgers, grilled steak . . . and many more.

5. **Is there an induction phase?**

No. The Belly Fat Cure is a lifestyle, which means that if it's not realistic for you from the very beginning, it will be tough to see it as a long-term plan. This doesn't mean that you won't see amazing results after only seven days. Several of my clients had weight loss in the double digits in the first week alone.

6. **Why don't I track proteins and fats on this plan?**

You won't be tracking proteins and fats because they don't directly affect the expansion of your waistline. Why? Various breakthrough studies done at Harvard University over the past decade have clearly shown that the main reason you have belly fat is because you've been eating too much of the *wrong* carbohydrates—sugar and processed carbohydrates—*not too much fat or protein.* It's that simple. You see, eating fats and proteins never significantly drives up the insulin level in your blood, which is the main way that your body likes to encourage the storage of fat— especially around your waistline. Bottom line: proteins and fat are processed by your body very differently. This is why the secret is to track just your sugar and carb intake. Does this mean that you can eat a whole cow or ten sticks of butter? No. You need to use common sense. But the good news is that proteins and fats satiate your hunger fast, so it's almost impossible to overeat them. And as you will see with all of my Carb Swap meals, my top pick for proteins is almost always a lean meat. And my top picks for fats come from egg yolks, raw butter, extra-virgin olive oil, flax oil, or fish oil.

7. **How long do I have to stay on this plan? Is there a different maintenance plan?**

Commit to one week and you'll see extraordinary results. Most of my clients are so thrilled that they plan to eat this way indefinitely. This is a lifestyle, not a diet, so there's no beginning and end phase. Once you start employing the Carb Swap System and the S/C Value, you'll get rid of your belly fat; plus, you'll feel revitalized, young, and ready for anything.

8. **Are there cheat days on this plan?**

No. Because this diet doesn't restrict anything—you can still eat all of your favorite foods—you won't need a cheat day.

9. **What do I do if I hit a plateau?**

Get back to basics and be diligent about tracking what you eat. If you do hit a weight-loss plateau, chances are you may not be sticking to exactly 15/6. Tracking what you eat each day will help keep you accountable and make sure that you're eating exactly what you need to maximize belly fat loss. Also, I recommend that you really pay attention to how much fiber you're getting each day—aim for 25 to 30 grams and you'll be amazed by how quickly your false belly fat disappears. Be sure to refer back to the chart on page 4; if you're near your goal weight, your weight loss will naturally slow down a bit.

10. **What exactly is a serving of a carbohydrate?**

With the S/C Value, one serving is anything that has 5 to 20 grams of carbohydrates; two servings is anything with 21 to 40 grams; three is anything with 41 to 60 grams. Remember, you get six servings of carbs throughout the day.

11. **Where can I look up the S/C Value of foods?**

Throughout the book, you'll find the S/C Value of all meals and food products pictured. You can also turn to Chapter 6 for the food list, which includes hundreds of other food items listed with their S/C Value.

12. **Can I be a vegan or vegetarian on this program?**

Yes. I've had several A-listers and other clients request vegan-friendly options for the Belly Fat Cure. The great news is that with just a few simple adaptations, you can eat to lose belly fat and stick to your vegan diet. Here's a quick "No-Excuses Day" customized for my vegan friends:

— Breakfast = Vega berry-flavored whole food health optimizer made with unsweetened almond milk or water

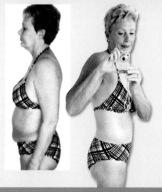

Patricia lost 20 pounds

Age: 66
Height: 5'7"
Pounds Lost: 20
Belly Inches Lost: 10

"For nearly 20 years of following every fad diet in the country, I tried unsuccessfully to lose 20 pounds. I'd come to believe that I was just too old to lose any weight . . . until I read about the Belly Fat Cure. This program is so easy to follow, and I was able to eat anything I wanted while following the S/C Value. I was never hungry, and it was amazing to watch the weight slip from my body. I am empowered by my beliefs and my actions to control my body. I am healthy and happy and have an enormous amount of energy to pursue my life goals."

BEST TIP FOR SUCCESS:

"Don't let yourself become hungry . . . eat all of your meals and snacks. You'll find that you won't crave the sweets if you're satisfied at meal times by eating foods on the program."

— Snack = 1 small handful of walnuts

— Lunch = 2 oz. El Burrito SoyTaco meatless filling on lettuce with cilantro, avocado, and red onion; topped with olive oil and vinegar

— Snack = 3 cubes of Vegan Gourmet mozzarella

— Dinner = It's All Good Meat-free Herb Dijon Breasts with sautéed green beans and ½ cup of brown rice

— Be sure to drink 8–10 glasses of water; and when you get a sweet craving, try my favorite Spry gum

You can also make a quick and easy scramble using tofu and El Burrito Soyrizo, which is a spicy meatless sausage—so good! Roll it up in a Tumaro's multigrain low-in-carbs tortilla with some vegan cheese and you've got a great meal with an S/C Value of 3/1. You can enjoy this for breakfast, lunch, or dinner.

There are so many great products out there (see page 303 for a list of meat-free options) these days that you can make a few adjustments in many of the Belly Fat Cure meals and enjoy them if you're a vegan or vegetarian. Try any of the Vega shakes for breakfast—most of them have just a 1/2 S/C Value and are loaded with protein and fiber. For lunch options, swap out any of the deli meats with Tofurky products and use Follow Your Heart Vegenaise (instead of mayonnaise) and mustard for a great sandwich. Try It's All Good "meats" for dinner dishes. For example, in the Sweet Pineapple Stir-Fry on page 221, use the beefless strips and you've got a tasty meat-free meal with the same S/C value of 5/2. Use Vegan Gourmet cheese for 0/0 snacks and in the Tasty Margherita Pizza (page 113). You can also make the Blueberry Velvet Muffins on page 81 using Bob's Red Mill Egg Replacer; top with Earth Balance original natural buttery spread.

13. **Can I do the Belly Fat Cure if I'm following a gluten-free diet?**
Yes. Since the program is based on a simple, clean way of eating, it can easily be adapted to be gluten free. Remember, we only track sugars and carbs, so I encourage you to eat plenty of lean proteins and healthy fats. My favorite gluten-free product (featured in the First-Class French Toast recipe on page 51) is the Light Brown Rice Loaf from Ener-G Foods. Check out **ener-g.com** for more on this bread and some of their other gluten-free products.

Here's a sample No-Excuses Day for gluten-free fans:

— Breakfast = 3 scrambled eggs with cheese and green onions, and a piece of light brown rice loaf with butter

- Snack = 1 small handful of walnuts

- Lunch = Turkey and Swiss on light brown rice loaf with mustard, mayo, and arugula

- Snack = 2 packages of string cheese

- Dinner = Grilled salmon with broccoli and Rice Expressions Organic Brown Rice Pilaf

- Enjoy a Zevia soda for a sweet treat during the day, and end your day with ½ cup blackberries with whipped cream (if you'd like dessert, that is).

It's simple, delicious eating that will help you lose belly fat quickly—without any gluten!

14. What if I'm pregnant?
If you are pregnant or breast-feeding, please check with your doctor before you begin our program.

15. Can my whole family follow this plan?
Yes! This plan will help adults of any age or gender lose belly fat. If you have kids who are overweight, I recommend consulting your doctor before starting them on the Belly Fat Cure. Reducing your kids' sugar intake will help keep them at a healthy weight, aid in focus (no sugar crashes in class!), and keep their immune systems strong. Many of the recipes in this book serve four—and the food is so delicious that you'll want to share it with your family.

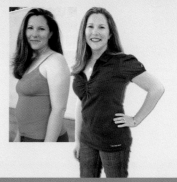

Patel lost 9 pounds

Age: 33
Height: 5'0"
Pounds Lost: 9
Belly Inches Lost: 2

"Once I started the Belly Fat Cure, I became accountable for everything I ate. I found that writing it all down was key. I started to read labels on everything I bought, and now I'm eating better and so is my family. I used to exercise for at least an hour three to four times a week and lost only five pounds. With this program, I didn't exercise—yet I lost nine pounds! I'm not an organized person, and even I can make this my lifestyle. For dessert, I have Clemmy's Chocolate Ice Cream four to five times a week. It's delicious!"

BEST TIP FOR SUCCESS:

"If you're on the run, grab a couple of tacos from Taco Bell. As for dinner, have something different every night so you enjoy the variety."

16. Where can I get success planners?

You can find a one-day planner at the end of Chapter 3 or visit **TheBellyFatCure.com** and join my free e-mail VIP club and get access to a PDF version.

17. Can I eat fewer than 15 sugars and 6 carbs every day?

You can certainly eat fewer than 15 grams of sugar a day, but you should try to have 6 servings of whole-grain carbs every day. If you're trying to accelerate your weight loss, I suggest eating all of your carbs before 3 P.M. (eat them with breakfast and lunch or as snacks, but not with dinner).

18. How much sugar can I eat and be safe?

I recommend that you eat no more than 15 grams of sugar a day; this is the ideal amount suggested for healthy weight and a strong immune system. You really can eat almost no sugar and be super healthy.

19. Is it possible to gain weight on this plan?

No, but note that if you add the Belly Fat Cure drink (page 101) to your diet and you aren't hydrated enough, you can accumulate false belly fat due to waste buildup. Wheat dextrin, which is found in Benefiber, is water-soluble fiber that will pull water from your body, so it's essential to stay well hydrated when you consume it. If you are drinking plenty of water and your elimination is still sluggish, your gut bacteria may be low (this is especially true if you've been taking antibiotics). The bacteria in your gut aid in peristalsis, which is the rhythmic contraction of the intestinal walls that literally keeps things moving. By simply adding a probiotic supplement to your diet, you can restore a healthy balance of beneficial bacteria that will make it easier for your body to clear the waste more efficiently. Also, be sure to get dietary fiber from other food sources such as brown rice, whole-wheat bread and crackers, and vegetables like artichokes and broccoli.

20. Are synthetic sugars bad?

Yes. I passionately suggest that you stay away from artificial sweeteners. The big three to avoid are: aspartame (NutraSweet and Equal), sucralose (Splenda), and saccharin (Sweet'N Low). These substances are known as excitotoxins, which means that they "overexcite" neurons in the brain, causing degeneration and even death in important nerve cells. When too many nerve cells die, your nervous system begins to malfunction, and it can't communicate with other parts of your body. This can ultimately lead to nervous-system disorders such as Parkinson's disease, multiple sclerosis, and Alzheimer's disease.

21. What are sugar alcohols, and do I have to count them?
Sugar alcohols don't actually contain any sugar or alcohol—they're a type of carbohydrate that requires little insulin to be converted to energy. They are used in foods for sweetness, but don't cause a significant spike in blood sugar or inhibit your immune system in any way. On the Belly Fat Cure, you won't be counting any grams listed as "sugar alcohols" in the sugar category; they may, however, be counted on a label under "total carbohydrates," which means that they will be counted as carbs on the S/C Value (but you won't have to track these separately).

22. I ate a sugar alcohol and got an upset stomach—is this normal?
Tolerance for sugar alcohols can vary from person to person. Moderate consumption of any sugar alcohol should cause no digestive issues, but excess consumption can lead to gas and bloating, so pay attention to your own personal level of tolerance. Research has shown that erythritol is the least likely to cause intestinal distress because it is almost completely absorbed by your small intestines and excreted in urine. If you prefer to use real sugar or honey, try to eat the raw varieties. Keep in mind that one teaspoon of sugar counts as 4 grams toward your daily 15, but one teaspoon of honey counts as 6 grams.

23. Is it true that I shouldn't give my dog xylitol or other sugar alcohols?
Xylitol has been linked to hypoglycemia and liver failure in dogs, but it hasn't been shown to have these effects in other species. Other sugar alcohols may cause diarrhea in dogs when consumed in excess, but they haven't been linked to more serious health problems. It's probably best to keep foods with sugar alcohols in them away from your pets—and be especially careful with xylitol around dogs.

24. Why won't I be tracking calories with the Belly Fat Cure?
Like with any plan, I recommend that you eat all things in moderation. However, I do not believe that counting calories is the most effective way to moderate your eating. Simply apply the S/C Value to your daily eating and you'll be successful in your weight loss and maintenance. You'll also notice that eating proteins, fats, and complex carbs will satiate you quicker and for longer periods of time, making overconsumption less likely.

25. Why is the S/C Value the same for different body sizes?
The S/C Value is designed to make sure that your body is keeping insulin low and producing the appetite-suppressing hormone leptin—no matter what your gender, age, or size—while also ensuring that you get enough servings of complex carbs a day. If you have a larger body type and feel that you need more food, you can try eating more protein, fats, or some of the lower-sugar vegetables. The goal is to follow the S/C Value and eat until you're satisfied within those requirements.

26. **Why can't I subtract the fiber carbs and use the net carbs as my carb intake?**
On the Belly Fat Cure, you'll be tracking sugar and carbs, not net carbs. One reason is for simplicity—many programs use a net carb system or they have you divide a fiber or sugar alcohol value in half, then subtract that from the total carb value . . . and I truly believe it makes things *too complicated*. This program is all about keeping it simple.

27. **How is this plan different from Atkins or the South Beach Diet?**
First of all, this is not a diet; this is a lifestyle. Plus, there is no extreme induction phase like in Atkins or South Beach—this is simply about making smarter choices from the beginning and sticking to it. You also won't be depriving yourself of any one thing. You've got to have a little sugar and some good carbs to stay satisfied and to really enjoy eating. My team and I are on the cutting edge and believe in smarter sweetness—you don't have to give up sweetness; you just have to be smart.

28. **Why do I count the sugars and carbs in fruits and vegetables?**
If your goal is truly to get rid of belly fat, then you have to stick to no more than 15 grams of sugar and be sure to eat 6 servings of carbs each day—this is from all food sources. Fructose, the sugar found in fruit, has specifically been linked to belly fat; since it goes directly to the liver to be processed, it gets converted to fat and leads to visceral belly fat and high cholesterol. Remember that fruit was created in tropical climates and in earlier times was available only certain times of the year—now we have access to everything, anytime, which is not how it was intended to be consumed. As for vegetables, even though they have nutrients, they're still carbohydrates that get converted to glucose and must be counted for belly fat loss. See my note on page 39 about adding fruit back into your diet after you reach your goal.

29. **Can I take prescription medications with the Belly Fat Cure drink?**
Wheat dextrin can interfere with the absorption of calcium, iron, zinc, and vitamin B_{12}; and may also affect anticoagulants, antidepressants, anti-gout agents, anti-inflammatory agents, diuretics, salicylates, tetracyclines, nitrofurantoin, insulin, lithium, and digoxin. I suggest taking medication or vitamins one hour before, or a few hours after, wheat dextrin to help prevent interactions. *To be safe, patients should be monitored for changes in medication requirements following the initiation of fiber therapy.*

30. **I have high blood pressure and/or high cholesterol and feel like I need to monitor my fat intake—can I still do this program?**
Yes, but I recommend that you speak with your doctor before starting any plan. Some research has shown that sugar is actually one of the biggest culprits when it comes to high cholesterol. Most sugars go directly to your liver and get converted to fat, which is sent into your blood, increasing your LDL, or bad cholesterol, levels. As for high blood pressure, one of the best things you can do for it is reduce your belly fat, which this program will do.

Selected Bibliography

Chapter 1

———. "Abdominal fat and what to do about it." *Harvard Women's Health Watch*. December 2006. **http://www.health .harvard.edu/newsweek/Abdominal-fat-and-what-to-do-about-it.htm.**

———. Mayo Clinic Staff. "Belly Fat in Women: How to Keep it Off." April 2007. **http://www.mayoclinic.com/health/ belly-fat/WO00128.**

Arver, S. "Testosterone and the Metabolic Syndrome." *Journal of Men's Health*. 5 (2008):S7–S10.

Escobar-Morreale, HF, JL San Millán. "Abdominal adiposity and the polycystic ovary syndrome." *Trends in Endocrinology & Metabolism*. 18 (2007):266–272.

Fontana L, JC Eagon, ME Trujillo, et al. "Visceral Fat Adipokine Secretion Is Associated With Systemic Inflammation in Obese Humans." *Diabetes*. 56 (2007):1010–1013.

Forouhi, NG, N Sattar, PM McKeigue. "Relation of C-reactive protein to body fat distribution and features of the metabolic syndrome in Europeans and South Asians." *International Journal of Obesity and Related Metabolic Disorders*. 25 (2001):1327–31.

Haffner SM, RA Valdez, MP Stern, et al. "Obesity, body fat distribution and sex hormones in men." *International Journal of Obesity and Related Metabolic Disorders*. 17 (1993):643–9.

Janssen, I, PT Katzmarzyk, R Ross. "Waist circumference and not body mass index explains obesity-related health risk." *American Journal of Clinical Nutrition*. 79 (2004):379–384.

Mah, PM, PM Wittert. "Obesity and testicular function." Uncorrected Proof. *Molecular and Cellular Endocrinology In Press*. Available online June 18, 2009.

Pischon T, H Boeing, K Hoffman, et al. "General and Abdominal Adiposity and Risk of Death in Europe." *The New England Journal of Medicine*. 359 (2008):2105–2120.

Rebuffé-Scrive M, P Mårin, P Björntorp. "Effect of testosterone on abdominal adipose tissue in men." *International Journal of Obesity*. 15 (1991):791–5.

Resnick, HE, EA Carter, M Aloia, et al. "Cross-sectional relationship of reported fatigue to obesity, diet, and physical activity: results from the third national health and nutrition examination survey." *Journal of Clinical Sleep Medicine*. 2 (2006):163–9.

Journal of Personal and Social Psychology. 65 (1993):293–307. Singh, D. "Adaptive Significance of Female Physical Attractiveness: Role of Waist-to-Hip Ratio."

Singh, D. "Waist-to-hip ratio and judgment of attractiveness and healthiness of female figures by male and female physicians." *International Journal of Obesity and Related Metabolic Disorders*. 18 (1994):731–7.

Vatanparast, H, PD Chilibeck, SM Cornish, et al. "DXA-derived Abdominal Fat Mass, Waist Circumference, and Blood Lipids in ostmenopausal Women." *Obesity.* (2009).

Vgontzas, AN, DA Papanicolaou, EO Bixler, et al. "Sleep Apnea and Daytime Sleepiness and Fatigue: Relation to Visceral Obesity, Insulin Resistance, and Hypercytokinemia." *The Journal of Clinical Endocrinology & Metabolism.* 85 (2000):1151–1158.

Wass P, U Waldenstrom, S Rossner, et al. "An android body fat distribution in females impairs the pregnancy rate of in-vitro fertilization-embryo transfer." *Human Reproduction.* 12 (1997):2057–2060.

Zhang C, KM Rexrode, RM van Dam, et al. "Abdominal obesity and the risk of all-cause, cardiovascular, and cancer mortality: sixteen years of follow-up in US women." *Circulation.* 117 (2008):1658–67.

Chapter 2

———. "Eat any sugar alcohol lately?" Yale-New Haven Nutrition Advisor. March 2005. **http://www.ynhh.com/online/nutrition/advisor/sugar_alcohol.html.**

Abou-Donia, MB, EM El-Masry, AA Abdel-Rahman, et al. "Splenda Alters Gut Microflora and Increases Intestinal P-Glycoprotein and Cytochrome P-450 in Male Rats." *Journal of Toxicology and Environmental Health.* Part A 71 (2008):1415–1429.

Arrigoni, E, F Brouns, R Amado. "Human gut microbiota does not ferment erythritol." *British Journal of Nutrition.* 94 (2005):643–646.

Barzilai, N, G Gupta. "Interaction between aging and syndrome X: new insights on the pathophysiology of fat distribution." *Annals of the New York Academy of Sciences.* 892 (1999):58–72.

Batterham, M, R Cavanagh, A Jenkins, et al. "High-protein meals may benefit fat oxidation and energy expenditure in individuals with higher body fat." *Nutrition & Dietetics.* 65 (2008):246–252.

Chan P, X Dy, JC Liu, et al. "The effect of stevioside on blood pressure and plasma catecholamines in spontaneously hypertensive rats." *Life Sciences.* 63 (1998):1679–84.

Clapp, R, D Davis, S Epstein, et al. "National Toxicology Program Board of Scientific Counselors' Report on Carcinogens Subcommittee." *CSPI Reports.* October 24, 1997.

Deardorff, J. "Agave provokes a bitter debate as a sweetener." *Chicago Tribune.* March 23, 2008.

Despres, JP, S Moorjani, PJ Lupien, et al. "Regional distribution of body fat, plasma lipoproteins, and cardiovascular disease." *Arteriosclerosis, Thrombosis, and Vascular Biology.* 10 (1990):497–511.

Falta, W. *Endocrine Diseases, Including Their Diagnosis and Treatment.* Philadelphia: P. Blakiston's Son & Co. 1923.

Fontana L, JC Eagon, ME Trujillo, et al. "Visceral Fat Adipokine Secretion Is Associated With Systemic Inflammation in Obese Humans." *Diabetes.* 56 (2007):1010–1013.

Gordon, ES, M Goldgerg, GJ Chosy. "A New Concept in the Treatment of Obesity." *The Journal of the American Medical Association.* 186 (1963):50–60.

Higginbotham, S, ZF Zhang, IM Lee, et al. "Dietary Glycemic Load and Risk of Colorectal Cancer in the Women's Health Study." *Journal of the National Cancer Institute.* 96 (2004):229–233.

Levi, B, MJ Werman. "Long-term fructose consumption accelerates glycation and several age-related variables in male rats." *The Journal of Nutrition.* 128 (1998):1442–9.

Liese, AD, M Schulz, F Fang, et al. "Dietary Glycemic Index and Glycemic Load, Carbohydrate and Fiber Intake, and Measures of Insulin Sensitivity, Secretion, and Adiposity in the Insulin Resistance Atherosclerosis Study." *Diabetes Care.* 28 (2005):2832–2838.

Liu G, CL Hughes, R Mathur, et al. "Metabolic effects of dietary lactose in adult female rats." *Reproduction Nutrition Development.* 2003 Nov-Dec;43 (6):567–76.

Maher, TJ, RJ Wurtmant. "Possible Neurologic Effects of Aspartame, a Widely Used Food Additive." *Environmental Health Perspectives.* 75 (1987):53–57.

Mattila, PT, M Knuuttila, LE Svanberg, et al. "Beneficial effects of dietary xylitol on mineralized and collagenous tissues." *Current Topics in Neutraceutical Research.* 1 (2003).

Newsholme, EA, C Start. *Regulation in Metabolism.* New York: John Wiley, 1973.

Olney JW, NB Farber, E Spitznagel, et al. "Increasing brain tumor rates: is there a link to aspartame?" *Journal of Neuropathology and Experimental Neurology.* 55 (1996):1115–23.

Passmore, R, YE Swindells. "Observations on the respiratory quotients and weight gain of man after eating large quantity of carbohydrate." *British Journal of Nutrition.* 17 (163):331–339.

Price, GM, CG Biava, BL Oser, et al. "Bladder Tumors in Rats Fed Cyclohexylamine or High Doses of a Mixture of Cyclamate and Saccharin." *Science.* 167 (1970):1131–1132.

Sanchez, A, Reeser, JL, Lau, HS, et al. "Role of sugars in human neutrophilic phagocytosis." *American Journal of Clinical Nutrition.* 26 (1973):1180–1184.

Savita, SM, K Sheela, S Sunanda, et al. "Health Implications of Stevia Rebaudiana." *Journal of Human Ecology.* 15 (2004):191–194.

Schulze, MB, JE Manson, D S Ludwig, et al. "Sugar-Sweetened Beverages, Weight Gain, and Incidence of Type 2 Diabetes in Young and Middle-Aged Women." *The Journal of the American Medical Association.* 292 (2004):927–934.

Singh, D. "Adaptive Significance of Female Physical Attractiveness: Role of Waist-to-Hip Ratio." *Journal of Personality and Social Psychology.* 65 (1993):293–307.

Singh, D. "Waist-to-hip ratio and judgment of attractiveness and healthiness of female figures by male and female physicians." *International Journal of Obesity and Related Metabolic Disorders.* 18 (1994):731–7.

Tavani, A, L Giordano, S Gallus, et al. C. "Consumption of sweet foods and breast cancer risk in Italy." *Annals of Oncology.* 17 (2006):341–345.

Vatanparast, H, PD Chilibeck, SM Cornish, et al. "DXA-derived Abdominal Fat Mass, Waist Circumference, and Blood Lipids in Postmenopausal Women." *Obesity.* (2009).

Vgontzas, AN, DA Papanicolaou, EO Bixler, et al. "Sleep Apnea and Daytime Sleepiness and Fatigue: Relation to Visceral Obesity, Insulin Resistance, and Hypercytokinemia." *The Journal of Clinical Endocrinology & Metabolism.* 85 (2000):1151–1158.

Walton RG, Hudak R, Green-Waite RJ. "Adverse reactions to aspartame: double-blind challenge in patients from a vulnerable population." *Biological Psychiatry.* 34 (1993):13–7.

Wass P, U Waldenstrom, S Rossner, et al. "An android body fat distribution in females impairs the pregnancy rate of in-vitro fertilization-embryo transfer." *Human Reproduction.* 12 (1997):2057–2060.

Yalow, RS, SA Berson. "Immunoassay of Endogenous Plasma Insulin in Man." *Journal of Clinical Investigation.* 39 (1960):1157–75.

Yalow, RS, SM Glick, J Roth, et. al. "Plasma Insulin and Growth Hormone Levels in Obesity and Diabetes." *Annals of the New York Academy of Sciences.* 131 (1965):357–73.

Zhang C, KM Rexrode, RM van Dam, et al. "Abdominal obesity and the risk of all-cause, cardiovascular, and cancer mortality: sixteen years of follow-up in US women." *Circulation.* 117 (2008):1658–67.

Additional Research

Barclay L. "Waist Girth Predicts Cardiovascular Risk Better Than BMI." *Medscape Medical News.* September 23, 2002.

Barzilai, N, J Wang, D Massilon, et al. "Leptin Selectively Decreases Visceral Adiposity and Enhances Insulin Action." *The Journal of Clinical Investigation.* 100 (1997):3105–3110.

Basciano H, L Federico, K Adeli, et al. "Fructose, insulin resistance, and metabolic dyslipidemia." *Nutrition & Metabolism.* 2 (2005):5.

Behan KJ, J Mbizo. "The Relationship Between Waist Circumference and Biomarkers for Diabetes and CVD in Healthy Non-Obese Women." *Laboratory Medicine.* 38 (2007):422–427.

Bergman RN, SP Kim, IR Hsu, et al. "Abdominal Obesity: Role in the Pathophysiology of Metabolic Disease and Cardiovascular Risk." *American Journal of Medicine.* 120 (2007):S3–S8.

Bergman RN, SP Kim, KJ Catalano, et al. "Why Visceral Fat is Bad: Mechanisms of the Metabolic Syndrome." *Obesity.* 14 (2006):16S–19S.

Beyer, PL, EM Caviar, and RW McCallum. "Fructose Intake at Current Levels in the United States May Cause Gastrointestinal Distress in Normal Adults." *Journal of the American Dietetic Association.* 105 (2005):1559–66.

Bjørbæk, C, BB Kahn. "Leptin Signaling in the Central Nervous System and the Periphery." *Recent Progress in Hormone Research*. 59 (2004):305–331.

Buss, D. "Strategies of Human Mating." *Psychological Topics*. 15 (2006):239–260.

Cleave TL. *The Saccharine Disease*. New Canaan, CT: Keats Publishing, August 1975.

Cohen, PG. "Obesity in men: The hypogonadal-estrogen receptor relationship and its effect on glucose homeostasis." *Medical Hypotheses*. 70 (2008):358–360.

Cordain L, SB Eaton, A Sebastian, et al. "Origins and evolution of the Western diet: health implications for the 21st century." *American Journal of Clinical Nutrition*. 81 (2005):341–354.

Costello, D. "The Price of Obesity." *Los Angeles Times*. April 1, 2005.

Demetra DC, PP Jones, AE Pimentel, et al. "Increased abdominal-to-peripheral fat distribution contributes to altered autonomic-circulatory control with human aging." *The American Journal of Physiology - Heart and Circulatory Physiology*. 287 (2004):H1530–H1537.

Diamant M, JL Hildo, MA van de Ree, et al. "The Association between Abdominal Visceral Fat and Carotid Stiffness Is Mediated by Circulating Inflammatory Markers in Uncomplicated Type 2 Diabetes." *The Journal of Clinical Endocrinology & Metabolism*. 90 (2005):1495–1501.

Ellwood M. "Fall's Fashion Makes the Waist More Important Than Ever." *New York Daily News*. October 4, 2007.

Fisher ML, M Voracek. "The shape of beauty: determinants of female physical attractiveness." *Journal of Cosmetic Dermatology*. 5 (2006):190–4.

Forouhi NG, N Sattar, PM McKeigu. "Relation of C-reactive protein to body fat distribution and features of the metabolic syndrome in Europeans and South Asians." *International Journal of Obesity*. 25 (2001):1327–1331.

Fung, TT, V Malik, KM Rexrode, et al. "Sweetened beverage consumption and risk of coronary heart disease in women." *American Journal of Clinical Nutrition*. 89 (2009):1037–1042.

Gosnell M. "Killer Fat." *Discover*. February 2007.

Hesketh, K, E Waters, J Green, et al. "Healthy Eating, activity and obesity prevention: a qualitative study of parent and child perceptions in Australia." *Health Promotion International*. 20 (2005):19–26.

Higginbotham, S, Z Zuo-Feng, L I-Min, et al. "Dietary Glycemic Load and Risk of Colorectal Cancer in the Women's Health." *Journal of the National Cancer Institute*. 96 (2004):229–233.

Katcher, HI, RS Legro, AR Kunselman, et al. "The Effects of a Whole Grain-Enriched Hypocaloric Diet on Cardiovascular Disease Risk Factors in Men and Women With Metabolic Syndrome." *American Journal of Clinical Nutrition*. 87 (2008):79–90.

Krajčovičová-Kudláčková, M, Kebeková, R Schinzel, et al. "Advanced Glycation End Products and Nutrition." *Physiology Research*. 51 (2002):313–316.

Mulligan, K, K Hootan, JM Schwarz, et al. "The Effects of Recombinant Human Leptin on Visceral Fat, Dyslipidemia, and Insulin Resistance in Patients with Human Immunodeficiency Virus-Associated Lipoatrophy and Hypoleptinemia." *Journal of Clinical Endocrinology & Metabolism.* 94 (2009):1137–1144.

Öhman MK, Y Shen, CI Obimba, et al. "Visceral Adipose Tissue Inflammation Accelerates Atherosclerosis in Apolipoprotein E–Deficient Mice." *Circulation.* 117 (2008):798–805.

Pagan, JA. and A Davila. "Obesity, Occupational Attainment, and Earnings." *Social Science Quarterly.* 78 (1997):756–70.

Pasquali, R. "Obesity, fat distribution and infertility." *Maturitas.* 54 (2006):363–371.

Reitzes, D. "Self and Health: Factors Influencing Self-Esteem and Functional Health." Paper presented at the annual meeting of the American Sociological Association, Marriott Hotel, Loews Philadelphia Hotel, Philadelphia, PA, Aug 12, 2005.

Rosch PJ. "All Obesity Is Not Created Equal." *Science.* 301 (2003):1325.

Sanches FMR, CM Avesani, MA Kamimura, et al. "Waist Circumference and Visceral Fat in CKD: A Cross-sectional Study." *American Journal of Kidney Diseases.* 52 (2008):66–73.

Stanhope, K, P Havel. "Fructose Consumption: Considerations for Future Research on Its Effects on Adipose Distribution, Lipid Metabolism, and Insulin Sensitivity in Humans." *The Journal of Nutrition.* 139 (2009):1236S–1241S.

Stanhope, KL, PJ Havel. "Fructose Consumption: Potential Mechanisms for its Effects to Increase Visceral Adiposity and Induce Dyslipidemia and Insulin Resistance." *Current Opinion in Lipidology.* 19 (2008):16–24.

Streeter SA, DH McBurney. "Waist-hip ratio and attractiveness. New evidence and a critique of 'a critical test.'" *Evolution and Human Behavior.* 24 (2003):88–98.

Teff, KL, SS Elliott, M Tschop, et al. "Dietary Fructose Reduces Circulating Insulin and Leptin, Attenuates Postprandial Suppression of Ghrelin, and Increases Triglycerides in Women." *The Journal of Clinical Endocrinology & Metabolism.* 89 (2004):2963–2972.

Tilg H, AR Moschen. "Adipocytokines: mediators linking adipose tissue, inflammation and immunity." *Nature Reviews Immunology.* 6 (2006)772–783.

Tracy RP. "Is Visceral Adiposity the 'Enemy Within'?" *Arteriosclerosis, Thrombosis, and Vascular Biology.* 21 (2001):881–883.

Wang Y, MA Beydoun, L Liang, et al. "Will all Americans become overweight or obese? Estimating the progression and cost of the US obesity epidemic." *Obesity.* 16 (2008):2323–30.

Whitaker, RC, JA Wright, MS Pepe, et al. "Predicting Obesity in Young Adulthood from Childhood and Parental Obesity." *The New England Journal of Medicine.* 337 (1997):869–873.

Zagorsky, JL. "Health and Wealth: The Late-20th Century Obesity Epidemic in the U.S." *Economics & Human Biology.* 3 (2005):296–313.

Zumoff B, GW Strain, LK Miller, et al. "Plasma free and non-sex-hormone-binding-globulin-bound testosterone are decreased in obese men in proportion to their degree of obesity." *Journal of Clinical Endocrinology & Metabolism.* 71 (1990):929–931.

Acknowledgments

To my dear wife, Heather, thank you for your endless support, magic, and love—I love you with all my heart. Thank you to my boys, Owen and Parker, for keeping me laughing and helping me taste all the yummy foods in this book. Thanks also to my dad, who helped me discover my true passion for health; and my grandmother Maria, whose independence and strength continue to amaze me.

My deepest gratitude to Carol Brooks, for your years of support and gratitude. A very special thank you to my invaluable circle of experts: Dr. Andrew Weil, Gary Taubes, Dr. Mehmet Oz, Dr. David Katz, Dr. James Novak, Dr. Terry Grossman, and Ray Kurzweil. I am lucky to have such renowned experts as mentors and friends.

To my clients—your support and efforts in helping me refine this program have truly been a gift. You are a critical part of creating the change . . . it all starts with you.

To Gretchen Lees and Jared Davis, my core content team—your hard work and incredible talent were invaluable to this project; I can't thank you enough for your dedication and commitment to creating truly outstanding content. Thank you to Michelle McGowen, for putting your passion for *The Belly Fat Cure* to work and for being a true asset to this project; and to Kim Barry, for all of the hours you dedicated. Thanks to Chance Miles for supporting our clients with knowledge and kindness. Extraordinary thanks to my culinary support team: Jeff Parker, Maria Sparks, Kim Werdenberg, Heather Henderson, Mark Lenos, and April Puda. Thank you to Lorraine E. Fisher for her excellent editorial eye, as well as Todd Brown for his help with our logo.

To Louise Hay, Reid Tracy, and the incredible support team at Hay House—you are passionate professionals who helped ensure the quality, integrity, and success of this book. Thank you to my media partners for helping me get my message out to the world: Brenda Turner and TJ Walter at *USA WEEKEND Magazine;* Ginnie Roeglin, Anita Thompson, David Fuller, and Tim Talevich at *The Coscto Connection;* Carol Brooks and Maggie Jaqua at *First for Women;* Jack Hogan, Laurie Berger, and Nicole McEwen at **LifeScript.com**; and Chad Hurley at **YouTube.com**.

To all of the amazing nutritional partners I've been so fortunate to connect with—I truly believe in the great products you're bringing to people, and I'm thrilled that you are part of the Belly Fat Cure Seal Program: Nathan Jones, Chuck Verde, Cynthia Davis, Gary Torres, Ira Laufer, Ken Probst, Kam Brown, Joseph Semprevivo, Steve Inglin, Kristen Livermore, Jay Robb, Derek and Jessica Newman, Ian Eisenberg, and Jon Gordon.

And a special thank you to my friends Bob Wietrak, Mary-Ellen Keating, Jade Beutler, Bruce Barlean, Richard Galanti, Debbie Ford, Joe Polish, Mike Koenings, Frank Kern, Anthony Robbins, Eben Pagan, Elliott Bisnow, Suzanne Somers, and Wayne Dyer.

Index of Recipes

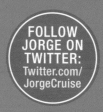

About the Author

JORGE CRUISE used to be 40 pounds overweight. Today, he is internationally recognized as the leading health expert for busy people and is the author of three consecutive *New York Times* best-selling series, with more than five million books in print in over 15 languages, including *8 Minutes in the Morning*® (HarperCollins), *The 3-Hour Diet*™ (HarperCollins), *The 12-Second Sequence*™ (Crown), and *Body at Home*™. He is also a contributing editor for *USA WEEKEND Magazine*, *The Costco Connection* magazine, *First for Women* magazine, and *Extra* TV. He has appeared on *The Oprah Winfrey Show*, CNN, *Good Morning America*, the *Today* show, *Dateline NBC*, *The View*, *The Tyra Banks Show,* and VH1.

Jorge received his bachelor's degree from the University of California, San Diego (UCSD); fitness credentials from the Cooper Institute for Aerobics Research, the American College of Sports Medicine (ACSM), and the American Council on Exercise (ACE).

Contact Jorge at: **JorgeCruise.com**. and follow him on-line at: **Twitter.com/JorgeCruise** and **YouTube.com/JorgeCruise**.

We hope you enjoyed this Hay House book. If you'd like to receive our online catalog featuring additional information on Hay House books and products, or if you'd like to find out more about the Hay Foundation, please contact:

Hay House, Inc., P.O. Box 5100, Carlsbad, CA 92018-5100

(760) 431-7695 or **(800) 654-5126**
(760) 431-6948 (fax) or **(800) 650-5115 (fax)**
www.hayhouse.com® • **www.hayfoundation.org**

• • •

Published and distributed in Australia by:
Hay House Australia Pty. Ltd., 18/36 Ralph St., Alexandria NSW 2015 •
Phone: 612-9669-4299 • *Fax:* 612-9669-4144 • www.hayhouse.com.au

Published and distributed in the United Kingdom by:
Hay House UK, Ltd., 292B Kensal Rd., London W10 5BE • *Phone:* 44-20-8962-1230 •
Fax: 44-20-8962-1239 • www.hayhouse.co.uk

Published and distributed in the Republic of South Africa by:
Hay House SA (Pty), Ltd., P.O. Box 990, Witkoppen 2068 • *Phone/Fax:* 27-11-467-8904 •
info@hayhouse.co.za • www.hayhouse.co.za

Published in India by:
Hay House Publishers India, Muskaan Complex, Plot No. 3, B-2, Vasant Kunj, New Delhi 110 070 •
Phone: 91-11-4176-1620 • *Fax:* 91-11-4176-1630 • www.hayhouse.co.in

Distributed in Canada by:
Raincoast, 9050 Shaughnessy St., Vancouver, B.C. V6P 6E5 •
Phone: (604) 323-7100 • *Fax:* (604) 323-2600 • www.raincoast.com

• • •

Take Your Soul on a Vacation

Visit **www.HealYourLife.com**® to regroup, recharge, and reconnect with your own magnificence.
Featuring blogs, mind-body-spirit news, and life-changing wisdom from Louise Hay and friends**.**

Visit **www.HealYourLife.com** today!

JOIN OUR FREE VIP E-MAIL CLUB!

Ensure your success with Jorge's FREE VIP e-mail club, and get immediate access to important updates, along with FREE video interviews with people such as Dr. Mehmet Oz and more.

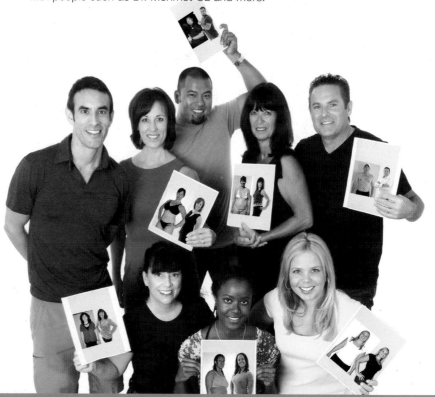

Vist **TheBellyFatCure.com**
and sign up for FREE today!